Testimonials

I want to share how much [Irini's] love, support and prayers helped me change my life. I have sold my house in a week and fell in love ... yes! And guess what, I have my kefi back! After so much pain it's nice to have some love in my life.
— Name withheld by request

Irini has helped me so much with making some major changes in my life. I had basically lost my kefi. I don't know how it happened but it did. I am educated, intelligent and a nice person but I was living with anxiety and fear, and of course this culminated in a depressing miserable life. I felt stuck, helpless and overwhelmed by fear. I was so unhappy. I couldn't see things changing. That's when Irini stepped in without judgement but with sensitivity, empathy and a positive and practical approach. She helped me focus on the future, making things good again, step by step. She believed in me when I didn't believe in myself. Irini has so much compassion and insight. She just gets it. Having Irini as a life coach was awesome.

I've made so many changes with Irini's help and God's Grace; I ended up selling my house without the enormous effort I thought I needed. I found a fantastic new place, joined a Greek dancing group and have pushed myself out of my comfort zone to do things I enjoy. I am so much happier now. I highly recommend Irini if you want to get your kefi back and create a happier and more enjoyable life.
— Haris Greek

Irini gently, but firmly, encouraged me to step out of my comfort zone and I'm truly grateful for her unwavering support. She has the knack

of knowing exactly what I've been putting off and pushing me to get it done. Her insistence on getting me on track and her unwavering faith in me has helped to get a number of programmes started. These programmes have ended up profiting me greatly and have inspired a lot of people in the process. I continue to enjoy working with Irini — she's intuitive, caring and respectful of the boundaries. If you want to make progress then Irini's your lady!
– Hayley Lowe, Internal Solutions

For quite some time I felt as though I wasn't happy with me. I had the best husband, great kids, good job and lovely home. Don't get me wrong, I was grateful for everything I had, but I wasn't happy with me. I knew I was living in fear and not achieving my dreams. I wanted to find my purpose.

I had known Irini for a long time but it was a mutual friend who brought us together a few years ago. I was instantly drawn to her kindness and her positive outlook. I knew I needed to fix the dysfunction I felt inside. I contacted Irini and started working with her. She was very insightful. I loved the fact she was a straight shooter but gentle when she needed to be. She challenged me while supporting me at the same time.

We did a lot of work together and now I have redefined my life. Through working with Irini, I realised I wanted to study further and be the best version of me, but also help others. I looked into further study and over time I would discuss my research with Irini. She was always encouraging and she helped to keep me focused and centred.

One day I found what I was looking for. I went back to university. Irini was one of the first people I told. She has backed me ever since. I had found my purpose studying psychological science. Without Irini's guidance I know I would still be searching. Thank you Irini xx
– Nicki Ottavi

Testimonials

Working through challenging times is always more possible when you have the presence of a skilled, mindful mentor. Enjoying the flow of life is also a richer experience with a mentor.
– Leah McKinnon, Educator

Irini has been absolutely amazing to work with.

Irini is the type of coach who understands and has 'been there, done that' – knowing that you cannot simply separate life and business, given that one impacts the other.
Irini has a gentle yet firm approach that gets results. I would recommend Irini to anyone.
– Kate Ryan-Taylor, Hippy Farm Girl

I felt that the process was non-threatening and simple, and allowed me to gain the confidence to begin my journey to find my kefi again. Irini enabled me to focus and to see my goals in a clear and simple way with excellent positive reinforcement. She took me deep enough and pushed me to think more about my situation, so I could achieve success.

I recommend anyone who needs some clarity about their life to spend some time with Irini either at a workshop or in a coaching session. She is awesome!
– Georgie Gregory

Irini has provided me with the confidence and passion to follow my heart and achieve my goals. Irini has a talent in bringing out the best in all of her clients. I am inspired by her passion and talent as well as her flexibility to adapt her style and techniques to many different situations. I have now reassessed my beliefs and values and have new tools and techniques, which have provided me with the motivation and clarity to achieve goals I never thought were possible.

Irini is excellent at [making] me really question my thinking, point of view, attitude, etc. She knows when to keep pushing me and when to persist with a line of questioning. Several times I had uncovered some meaningful insights but Irini would continue with a confronting line of questioning ... eventually I would break through a mental barrier and get a significant shift in thinking.

Irini has provided valuable coaching in a variety of personal and work life areas. From a recent session where she assisted me with a planning method to help me decide my career direction, to gaining clarity in what is important to me in my life and where to put my focus.
— *Tanya Stephenson, The Grief Recovery Specialist*

I have worked with Irini for the past year and I feel extremely privileged to have her as a coach. I now have the tools I need to take actions that maximise results in my business.

Through working with Irini I have been able to improve the quality of clients as well as how much they pay me. She helped me prioritise what was important in my professional life. Her coaching was the start of my journey into a confident leadership position within my business. Irini is able to strike a unique balance of careful listening as she confidently shares her wealth of experience and ideas. She quickly pinpoints the crux of a situation and gives me helpful insights. She has helped me develop ways to deal with situations using my own knowledge and self-awareness. I have come to regard Irini as a valued friend as well as business advisor.
— *Georgie Fitzgerald, CEO, Georgie Heart Media*

The Kefi Effect

Busting the Myth of the Good Greek Girl

Irini Kalis

First published by Busybird Publishing 2018
Copyright © 2018 Irini Kalis

ISBN
Print: 978-1-925692-96-9
Ebook: 978-1-925692-49-5

Irini Kalis has asserted her right under the Copyright, Designs and Patents Act 1988 to be identified as the author of this work. The information in this book is based on the author's experiences and opinions. The publisher specifically disclaims responsibility for any adverse consequences, which may result from use of the information contained herein. Permission to use information has been sought by the author. Any breaches will be rectified in further editions of the book.

All rights reserved. No part of this publication may be reproduced, stored in or introduced into a retrieval system, or transmitted in any form, or by any means (electronic, mechanical, photocopying, recording or otherwise) without the prior written permission of the author. Any person who does any unauthorised act in relation to this publication may be liable to criminal prosecution and civil claims for damages. Enquiries should be made through the publisher.

Cover image: Kev Howlett
Cover design: Busybird Publishing
Layout and typesetting: WorkingType www.workingtype.com.au

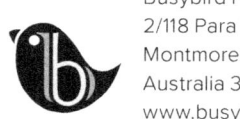

Busybird Publishing
2/118 Para Road
Montmorency, Victoria
Australia 3094
www.busybird.com.au

Dedication

I dedicate my book firstly to my gorgeous kids Andrew and Katina: you are my why. I needed to get my kefi back so you could live amazing kefi-filled lives.

Secondly, to my mum and dad who would be so proud of this work – they taught me all I know about how to serve others, to give my all, to expect the best of myself and to love my Greek heritage.

Lastly, to all the women of Greek heritage out there who just need a little kefi in their life – this is for you.

Contents

Introduction		1
Chapter 1	*Kefi Reality*	9
Chapter 2	*Kefi What*	21
Chapter 3	*Kefi Chick*	35
Chapter 4	*Kefi Family*	49
Chapter 5	*Kefi Friends*	61
Chapter 6	*Kefi Future*	73
Chapter 7	*Kefi Fortune*	85
Chapter 8	*Kefi Faith*	97
Chapter 9	*Kefi Fit*	111
Chapter 10	*Kefi Feast*	123
Chapter 11	*Kefi Flame*	135
Chapter 12	*Kefi Life*	147
Afterword		157
Glossary		159
Appendix 1 – *Budget Template*		161
Appendix 2 – *SMART Goals Template*		163
About the Author		165
Kefi Bonus		167
The Kefi Effect – *Opportunities and Programs*		169

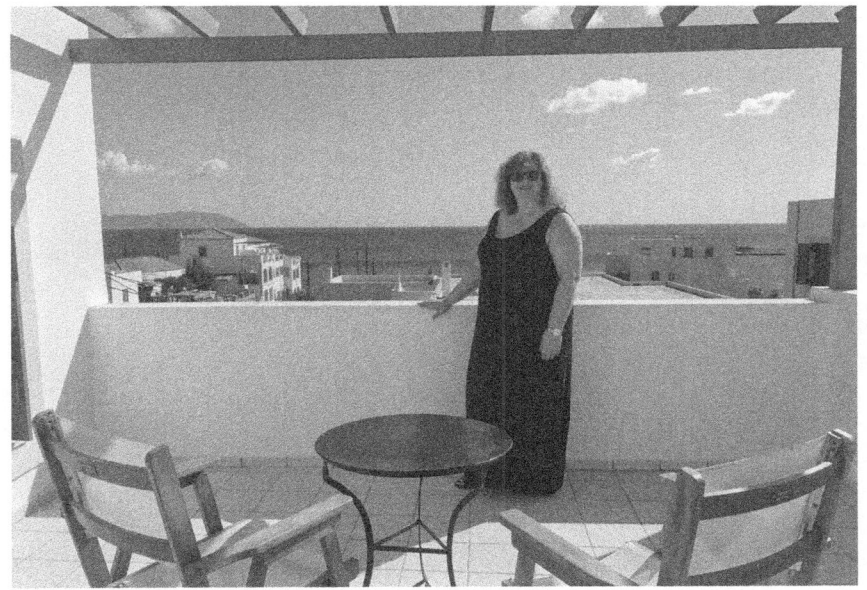

Introduction

A Dedication – I see you!

You are amazing.
I can see you when you think no one can.
I sense your pain,
the loss of the parts of you that matter.
You are whole, every piece of you is intact.
It is hard for you to see YOU!
You are kind.
You are loving.
You are beautiful.
You matter!
Raise your eyes from looking down.
So you haven't achieved those goals ... yet.
You are carrying around the shame and the guilt ...
Those extra kilos that have kept piling on.
Hanging on to the pain, the hurt keeping safe.
You are still that amazing, creative, loving woman you always were.
In your heart you are a passionate woman who knows what she wants.
You haven't quite worked out how.
You have forgotten to give yourself permission.
To ask for what you want.
To ask yourself first.
How would you like your life to be? Now go take that step towards that brilliant life!
Life starts with YOU!

I am the Kefi Chick, and it has taken me quite a few years to get to where I am today. I am an ordinary woman of Greek origin, born in Australia with a deep love of all things Greek — well, most things in any case.

Life is a journey, as we are so often told. At times I felt I could bear no more pain, hurt or suffering, with things not going my way and blaming others for my lot. I lost myself somewhere between my teenage years, working as a teacher from my early twenties until my forties when I was a wife and a mother who had lost all confidence, self-esteem and hope. I was living a life without kefi.

Growing up Greek is different for my kids than when it was for me and my siblings. How do I start to make sense of how I grew up, ending up lost and alone in adulthood? Fast forward to now, where I have accumulated understandings and teachings over time, providing me with a bank of wisdom to draw on to help others like you. Growing up Greek came with rules; there was an unwritten code of conduct and a belief system that didn't match that of my non-Greek friends. 'What will people say?' was a popular phrase that came from mothers, fathers, grandparents, aunts and uncles; it was often enough to prevent non-approved activities.

It wasn't that many years ago when someone asked me about my life dreams. Dreams? What are they? You mean I can look ahead and work towards the things I want for myself? I had no understanding that I could have hopes and aspirations just for me! I had no idea how to answer this person who had for three hours eloquently and explicitly shared his dreams.

I realised that I had been going through life's motions; I felt I wasn't worthy of having dreams and that I should be satisfied

Introduction

with the life I already had. I should be content with being a school teacher for the rest of my life, not having satisfying relationships, beating myself up and feeling unfulfilled. I knew something was missing in my life. I had started thinking about myself in the third person.

This conversation-starter about hopes and dreams happened a short while after my I had separated from my Aussie husband, who is a good man, just not the ideal one for me. A tiny candle had been lit but I just couldn't see the light yet. I had been so immersed in feeling negative about myself and the world around me that I couldn't *see*. I had thought I was travelling okay. Time is a wonderful teacher – I now know that life back then was devoid of kefi.

No kefi existed in my life anywhere. I hung around people I thought were uplifting – in fact they drained me and distracted me from feeling the emotions I needed to feel. I bottled up grief from when my dad died when I was 13, painful relationships, divorce, issues in the workplace, bullying, friendship battles and so on. As a Good Greek Girl I never expected to get divorced; marriage is forever, so you are expected to weather the storm and put up with it. As a Good Greek Girl I avoided conflict and became the pick-me girl. Every time there was a job to do or extra duties in the school where I worked, I would put my hand up. I would overload myself and then crash and burn later.

A Good Greek Girl does not abandon a well paying job! Teaching is one of the family professions – several of us are good at it, we have a talent for it. I was a teacher for twenty-four years, when in 2010 I decided to give it all up – it felt meaningless and unfulfilling on so many levels. In my early years, I loved it when a teacher had control over curriculum and could engage students in ways which empowered them as learners.

It took a few more years before I was to fully comprehend my true calling, and to unpack how to assist the most people possible. My mother's father came to Australia in 1905 from the Ionian island of Kythera. My *papou*'s energy was in his entrepreneurial acumen and ability. He was credited with the term 'the Casimaty Touch' — a bit like the Midas Touch. It's how I came to coin 'the Kefi Touch', which is about all that I do in all areas of my life to bring a little bit of kefi and happiness.

My inspiration to embrace the word kefi came from two events. The first was when I went to a Hay House event and one of the speakers spoke about the word 'kefi'. I asked myself, 'How can a non-Greek person claim this word which is ours?' She had everyone up dancing and having a great time. Almost instantly I thought, *Wow — I could do that!*

The second moment of inspiration was when I watched the Nia Vardalos movie *My Life in Ruins*. The female lead is a tour guide waiting to get her real job at a university, but in the meantime she has a summer job. She has no kefi and finds it difficult to connect with the tourists on her bus. It is about her journey as she reclaims her kefi and relationships with the people on the bus. Life turns around in a mighty big way!

Life changes on so many levels when you have your kefi — you love life and you're filled with an innate joy and vitality that is infectious. People are drawn to you and you love living your fulfilling and enriching life. Bad stuff still happens, but you've learnt the art of picking yourself up and dusting yourself off in an instant — or at least pretty quickly!

Introduction

I may not have been a tour guide on a bus, but there are some remarkable similarities with *My Life in Ruins* in the way I live my life now compared with about ten years ago. What I learnt is that it is okay to be vulnerable and to feel all of my feelings. I released my need to control everything all of the time, in favour of being the real authentic me – because I liked that me. I found my motivation to get things done, to take risks, to take the plunge doing the things I always dreamt of. I took responsibility for me.

If you ask yourself how you'll ever get over death, loss, tragedy, trauma, or crisis, I am here to share with you that it is possible to feel different, to re-emerge from the shadows whole and fulfilled. You can deal with people who trigger you or make you feel you are not good enough. You can heal and get past this dark place.

You may feel life is too hard: dysfunctional relationships hamper you, you overeat, a perfect life is out of reach, you are tired of everything and are looking for a magic spell to pull you out of your dreary life. You have stopped taking care of yourself or feel life is a façade; you go through the motions like a zombie. No one gets you, no one cares – everyone has unrealistic expectations of you, so you feel like you are caring and giving to everyone else and there is nothing left in the tank for you.

You are stuck in a life which is not what you imagined it to be.

The Kefi Effect is reaching out to you, calling to you. Take the outstretched hand offered here. Here you will find what you need to strengthen yourself and move away from being undermined by fear and despair. Move towards compassion and radiance – allow transformation to happen, in order to heal and feel whole again. Let your kefi shine!

Rejoice in your heritage, culture and traditions as you become more acquainted with your identity. Celebrate the great in you that is itching to be revealed.

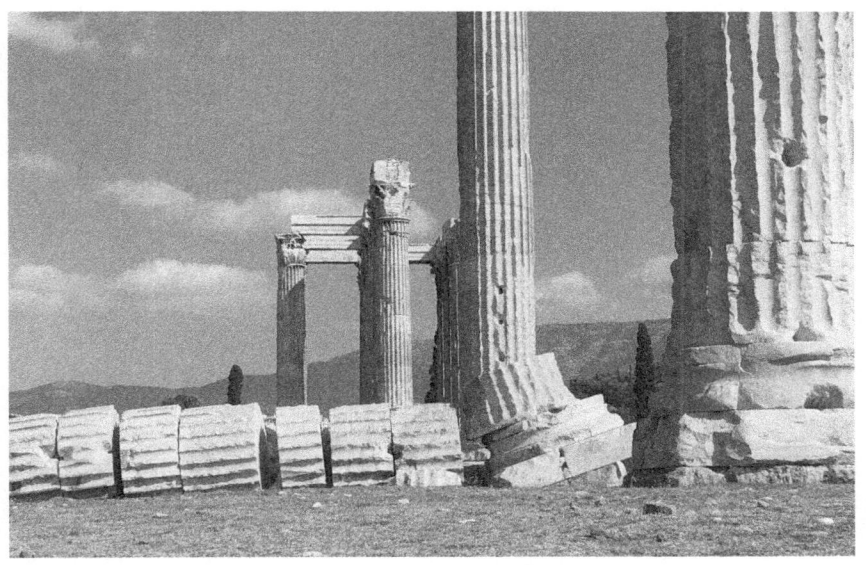

Chapter 1

Kefi Reality

'You don't develop courage by being happy in your relationships every day. You develop it by surviving difficult times and challenging adversity.'
– **Epicurus, philosopher**

'Since we cannot change reality, let us change the eyes which see reality.'
– **Nikos Kazantzakis, writer**

The reality is that it can be tough getting over stuff. We make excuses to keep ourselves small and safe, to not rock the boat or attract attention to ourselves. Who wants to get out there and expose themselves to all that discomfort and stress, where criticism, judgement and gossip live?

Imagine a life where kefi feels easy and stress-free — where it flows and you deal with whatever life throws at you effortlessly. One word can help you change your world. Wouldn't it be great to be able to learn from someone who gets it? Someone who's been through the tough stuff and has come out the other side to make it easier for people to follow behind?

Your mission, should you choose to accept it, is to learn implementable and simple strategies that I know work, some things that sometimes can be hard and sometimes can be easy. What starts off as hard becomes easy. Things can click quickly as you build momentum and make choices which have a big collective impact! The end result will be the same: you'll get your kefi back and you'll be able to live the life that you've always dreamed of, get stuff done and be happy.

'Kefi' is a four letter Greek word which packs a great deal of punch! It can have an immense impact on all areas of your life.

Isn't it time to give yourself permission to be that person who is going to be able to find your kefi and get stuff done? Get everything done that you keep talking about and planning to do. The things that you always dream of, the things that you always want to have, but you think are just out of your reach. The things you have been conditioned to think you are not worthy of.

Imagine your life in a few months' time – in one, five or ten years. Are you going to look back and wish you'd done something differently? Will you see the rewards of the work you have done? Will you feel happy with who and what you'll see as you look back on your life? Are you going to be able to say you did all that you could, that you wanted? Or will you have regrets that you didn't take the big action to be healthier, or spend time with the people you love telling them so? Will you have loved someone with all of your heart? Will you have given yourself to the people who are important in your life and will you have contributed to them reaching their potential?

The reality is that to have a happy, kefi-filled life, you need to take some action. Some work on your part is required to disrupt the more problematic things that you have learnt in your Greek family, or your Italian family, or any other culture that you have as your background.

Sometimes getting things done creates feelings of discomfort; you will need to commit to getting comfortable with feeling uncomfortable. When you embrace your fear of change and you get on with it, this is where your circumstances will change. You take small steps, even baby steps towards something you never thought possible, and in that space you will surprise yourself.

When a Greek person mentions the word kefi, they know instantly that they are referring to feelings of joy, enjoyment, passion, happiness and excitement. It means having fun and loving life. A Greek knows what that feeling is and can identify when they have it in an instant.

The problem is, it's really hard to actually define the word in English, because there is really nothing that comes close to the feeling of kefi. It's really more about experiencing something positive. The real benefit of finding your kefi, however, is finding that when times aren't good, you can pick yourself up and come out the other side. When things are going well, everyone has their kefi. But what do you do when things aren't going so well?

Many people think kefi is just about being the life of the party; it is so much more than that. It embodies everything — your whole body, mind and soul. It has an impact on your self-talk, your inner critic, how you participate in life and how you react to others, especially when things go wrong.

Having kefi is empowering; it impacts on how you relate to the people in your life on a day to day basis and you feel free to be yourself. To be clear, it is not about being the life of the party. It is about being the life of your own party! To be the real authentic *you* all of the time. To make decisions and choices that you wish to make, not the ones you think will make you popular with friends and family. To enjoy the fruits of your labour in all areas of your life. To live a life filled with passion as you do the things you love with the people that you love — and most importantly, you pay it forward!

I can tell you that there's been many times in the past when I just couldn't get myself moving. I was stuck, feeling depressed — what was I going to do to get out of this funk? I would overthink and overdramatise things — I was unable to get out of the rut. I played the blame game, the one where I didn't take personal responsibility. That is, until I started working on myself and exploring the personal development world. More about that a bit later.

If you had a crystal ball and you could look into the future, what do you want to see? Will you have an amazing house? Will you be on holiday? Will you have lots of people around you? Will you feel fulfilled? Will you feel yourself without those negative thoughts that keep going on and on and on? Will you hear the love in other people's voices as they're talking to you?

So how do you get all of this?

Follow the steps in this book; taking it on board and deciding it is possible is the very first thing you can do for you. Maybe you have several areas of your life in order and there are few things you can work on right now to make a difference.

Just stop for a moment and imagine how you want it to be. What do you see and hear? How do you feel and how do you think about things? Is it different to the life that you're currently living? What could you do differently to change it up? What do you need to do? It's quite simple really: as soon as you find that kefi, you're going to be on the road to where you want to be.

Quite often when I'm talking to people, they tell me it's hard to change. Well, it's only hard when it's foreign and new, so when you don't know what it is that you want to change, the common answer is 'it's too hard'. In reality, change can happen in an instant. You can choose to change right now in this very moment and leave the shell of the person who is walking through life like a zombie, carrying those experiences of divorce, death in the family, career issues, bullying – and that's only the start of the things that you may have experienced.

All of those things define who you are, and it's allowing them to influence what you do and how you behave today or you chalk that up to experience, see it as a lesson and you say, 'Okay, I'm going to move on and change the way that I experience life.'

Change is simple when you choose it.

My story includes many of those things. I was a Good Greek Girl who got married to a man who was not Greek; we did not get married in the Greek church, much to my mother's disappointment. It was immediately clear that our values were not aligned and we ended up clashing over the small stuff.

Now that I understand my values, I can see that our belief systems were totally different and no middle ground could be found. The way that we experience family, and the way we behave and do things, are really different from one another. We grew up in Australian households with different experiences and ways of being. We didn't really have the same background, the same cultural understanding, the same traditions — all of those things that come from having your heritage. I learnt from this time of my life that knowing what you believe in and what is important is essential.

I'm not saying that my ex-husband was a bad man — that is not true. And there have been bonuses: my children and the friendship I retained with my-in-laws. But when it came to our relationship, my expectations of how life would be in marriage were very different to the reality. The bottom line was that we just weren't compatible. I found that it was really easy to let go, once I understood that the relationship was not what I needed to make myself whole — in no way did it bring out my potential and in no way did I contribute to his potential as well.

Life sometimes doesn't go the way that you want it to. When I got married, I did think it was going to be for life – just like I thought I had selected a career for life in teaching. 'Teaching is a good profession for women,' I heard over and over. I never thought I would double in size and would not be a slim person. I never thought I would experience so many of the things I have.

Sometimes the more you focus on something that doesn't work out, the longer you'll feel let down. When I concentrated on the negative components of my marriage, my career and the things that didn't go right, it was really heavy. I spent my life in the pantry, putting more and more weight on. And I have been challenged for many years to shift that weight.

What happens when life doesn't work out the way you want it to? Sometimes the promotion doesn't pan out. Who cares in the end? Only you. There was a time when I aspired to be a school principal. The process was to become a senior teacher, an assistant principal and then a principal. Along the way I applied for several jobs; it was a real blow to my ego when life didn't go the way that I wanted it to. I didn't crack the promotions, I didn't get picked. I felt like I was back at school, being picked last to join a team during sport.

I am sure you have your own stories; for now let's just focus on the simple things, and understand what kefi is. Know that it's possible to change and possible to influence the world around you.

Overall you can see that kefi is simply a word for experiencing something positive. The real benefit of finding your kefi, however, is to keep you afloat when things aren't at their best or when things are challenging you, and it's really easy to spiral down into negativity.

Let's focus on what you could do, how you want to feel and where you're going to go with it all.

Sometimes you have to give change a chance. I'm here to tell you, when you get over yourself, change can be really easy and sometimes it's about understanding the steps. Change doesn't have to be a big monumental 'wipe the slate clean' process. Sometimes it can be simple things. A small step in clearing the clutter in your zone, one room at a time. Introducing one new exercise behaviour. Changing your diet slightly. Surrounding yourself with uplifting people.

Those are the sorts of things that I've found have made a significant difference in my life.

Sometimes it's easy to see that everything's a mess in your home, but you can't see how to clear your clutter. 'Clutter' is an indication that things aren't right on the inside of yourself – the outside can often be a reflection. You can stay stagnant or you can invest in yourself. It's not about how much money you've got or employing coaches who are really expensive – it's about spending the time. It will make a difference if you can take simple steps, such as reading this book right through to the end – implement what works for you, and one day you'll stop and observe for yourself how things have changed.

Personal experience has taught me that if you just keep going and keep trying new things, you will eventually find something that works for you.

There is no 'one size fits all' strategy or philosophy. Sometimes people believe that one thing will make the difference and voila, life will be beautiful. People think that what they see is someone else having a charmed life. It isn't always like that. At times they have a wall around them, hiding the real truth. Other people just get on with life, take it on the chin and move on.

Stepping out and trying something new, taking a risk, can be the issue. There's a great saying: 'feel the fear and do it anyway'. When I embraced that, I found that I could achieve just about anything. I used to think that I was a very quiet person and quite often I would never say what I wanted to say, because I was exceptionally afraid of confrontation. What I learnt along the way is that when I confronted people, when I said what I needed to say for me, then new opportunities opened up. Quite often, the whole relationship changed dramatically. It can be a really wonderful thing when you see what happens.

When you understand who you are, what you believe in and traditions, culture and heritage, then you have a huge sense of identity. Your sense of identity is where it all comes into play.

A Good Greek Girl knows who she is and understands the way things work. However, sometimes the way things work can exploit your perfectionist tendencies or your inability to say no to something. You keep saying yes to doing things and overloading yourself — or you do the opposite and you become the rebel, damaging relationships around you rather than understanding what you need to do for yourself. Empowering yourself along the way will give you so much freedom and inspire you to be more.

As an Australian woman of Greek decent there is so much that creates confusion. On the one hand, we are surrounded by the social morays of the family and society; and on the other hand, it is about finding our way in the world while keeping safe. Getting out of the Good Greek Girl comfort zone can be quite a challenge — and yet when it becomes possible and a new world is opened up, it can feel like it is impossible to please everyone. Pleasing yourself first, as long as it does not harm others, is the first understanding that will enable your kefi. Honouring your personal beliefs and values in the context of maintaining your safety net and how you fit into the world around you plays a substantial role in understanding and maintaining a kefi life.

I know for a fact that when I married my husband, he was not from my tribe, my community, my culture — he was not from where I came from. He didn't quite get it. I know that whilst there were times when things were great, the actual big picture stuff just didn't happen the way it needed to for me.

What I would suggest to you that if you're in any relationship including with friends, if the people aren't from your tribe, because you don't have anything in common that you share, then often there's a mismatch.

Quite a lot of people say to me, 'I keep getting picked on by everyone and they just don't get me.'

Well, sometimes that feeling of being bullied can start with yourself. If you don't *get* yourself, how could anyone else get you? You can be positive, embrace your culture and follow through with the things that you say you're going to do. So instead of having lots of UFOs (unfinished objects) in your world, you'll find that things are really successful.

As you complete the audit of your life and where you would like to add more kefi, you will gain the clarity you are looking for.

Three action steps you can take to increase your kefi:

1) Take a walk through your family history. When did your family leave Greece (or another country of origin), where did they leave from and where did they come to? Know your family story so you understand your identity. Look through old family photo albums or talk to your grandparents and parents about what they know.

2) Create your vision of how you would like your life to be. Focus on what you will see, hear, think and feel in the life you are creating for yourself. Believe that it is possible. This can be done by writing it all down, by creating a vision board or mind map.

3) Every day spend time writing a 'Brain Dump'. Let it all out, write about whatever comes into your head. Set the timer for 10–15 minutes and just write. There is no right or wrong way to do this exercise. It will assist you clear the overthinking and lack of clarity.

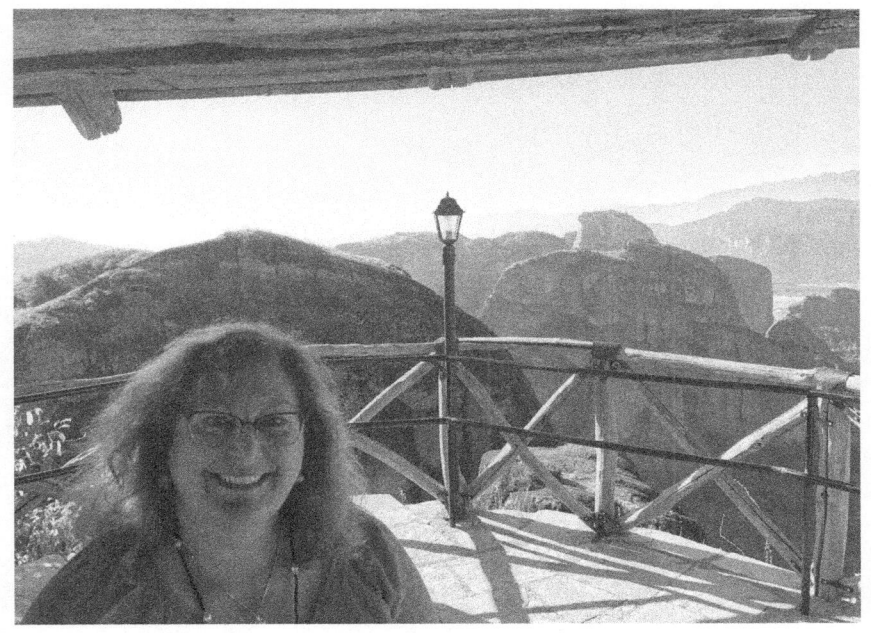

Chapter 2

Kefi What

'Happiness depends upon ourselves.'
— **Aristotle, philosopher**

'The secret of happiness is freedom ... and the secret of freedom is courage.'
— **Thucydides, historian**

The ultimate goal of being human is the desire to be happy. With kefi in your life, it is possible to get a whole lot closer to that goal. Everybody (and I mean everybody) wants to be happy. That is one of our core desires: the thing that everybody craves, that we work towards for ourselves, our children, our families and our friends. At the core of happiness is kefi: the feeling that contributes to a positive thinking way of life.

Essential to this concept of happiness is an understanding of what happiness looks like for each individual. Is it all about a state of mind, a feeling in your heart. How do you know when happiness kicks in? What rules do you have for happiness? Often the focus is more on what it is not, and the negative emotional state from a sense of 'lack'; these are so much easier to identify.

But how do you get that to happen when things aren't going quite the way that you want them to? At those times you may feel like you are drowning in doubt, lack and negativity.

For a long time now, I have been striving to become happy again. I remember being unhappy when my Dad died when I was thirteen, or perhaps even younger when my parents went into a shop when I was three and they were busy working – I can't really pinpoint it exactly, I just know there was a time in my life when I didn't feel joy, safety, empowerment, freedom, inspiration or kindness to myself and others. I spent a lot of time in my head, creating scenarios and overthinking rather than living in the now!

Step by step and little by little, I've gotten to where I need to be. Yes, there are still some things that I'm working on, but I'm a work in progress, as you can imagine. Life is all about learning and sometimes you can't learn it all in one go.

Do you really want to live a life of being envious, unfulfilled, depressed and heavy? Do you want to always feel attacked by people and that you're never good enough? Where your self-esteem is really low and you have no idea who you are and what you want?

When you embrace your traditions, culture and heritage, it's the start of the healing process. You recognise and acknowledge who you are and what you know to be true for you by going back to your roots and looking at how it all evolved — by seeing how your family came to be here living in Australia, or America, or Canada, or anywhere else in the world.

The journey that those family members took to get to where we are now is huge. It is essential to honour your roots, to know why they came to leave their homeland and the impact of where your family fits now.

My family on my mother's side came from the small Ionian island of Kythera, at the base of the Peloponnese. In 1905 my grandfather was sent by his dad to come to Australia. Great-grandfather George had already spent some time in Australia from 1891 to 1896. Times were tough in Greece and the family was struggling. There was not enough to eat and so it was time for my grandfather to come to a new country, to forge a new life for his family.

My grandfather was fourteen at the time and he got his first pair of shoes. His first job was as a kitchenhand at the Acropolis Café

Chapter 2   Kefi What

in Sydney for five shillings a week. He spent some time working in the fishing industry and in the fish market.

My family ended up in Hobart, Tasmania, only because my grandfather came to have a look around in 1914 on boat on the *Paloona*, as that was the only means of transport at the time. He decided that Hobart was a quiet town and therefore was not for him, so he thought that he'd head back to Sydney (the 'big smoke'). The Union Steamship Company was closed for the weekend and he couldn't organise his return to Sydney. In the meantime, what do you do? You buy a business and decide to stay. That's how Mum's family ended up staying in Hobart.

In 1929, he went back to Kythera; he was thirty-eight at the time and he married my eighteen year old grandmother. She was to become the powerhouse of the family with six children and seventeen grandchildren. Her hospitality and her cooking skills are legendary and have been passed on down the line. Coming to Australia, she found quite a new world.

My father's side of the family, on the other hand: Dad came in 1956 on an assisted passage at the age of 18, a bit like the ten pound Pom program, but he came from Greece. He spent some time at Bonegilla, and cutting sugar cane in north Queensland. He did other jobs until he arrived in Hobart, and that's where Mum and Dad met – and the rest is history. They ended up in a corner store in 1967 and we lived above the shop. We lived there until 1978 when we left because Dad got sick.

Most people have a similar story. Some of my friends have a story where their parents got married by proxy: the wife travelled to Australia without having met the husband, who then went to the airport or the boat with a photograph so he could recognise his new wife. Those stories are quite common.

When you know who you are and where you've come from, it gives you a true sense of identity. It really helps you become that person you want to be. You have to understand who you are before you can go through the big healing process.

You want to be able to lift up your spirit. You want to be able to strengthen those pillars, as they are the foundations of the Columns of Strength. The four pillars are kindness, empowerment, freedom and inspiration. They make up the letters of the word 'kefi'.

- **Kindness** is so important, it's the number one pillar for kefi. It's how you treat yourself. So often my clients talk about the bullies in their lives – they get a shock when they realise the worst bully is themselves.

- Secondly, you need to be able to **empower** yourself. Being able to achieve and do what you can because you choose to do so is powerful. It is where your inner strength and courage come from when times are tough, when it is time to stand up and be counted, when the answer is no.

- Thirdly, you need to be able to find **freedom** for yourself to be who you are, and not being governed by someone else's rules and expectations.

- Lastly, **inspiration** is when you live an inspired life: life is wonderful and easy, and it appears as if you live a charmed life. That's what you're aiming for; that's what happiness is.

The majority of women won't act on their dreams, instead putting up with a mediocre life full of regrets. The Good Greek Girl is ingrained in such a way that it is a challenge to break free and select the parts you believe are worth celebrating and holding on to. Being a Good Greek Girl isn't always bad – it just depends who is ruling your thinking and behaviour. It's about valuing the good parts and blending them with what you want for yourself.

I talk to women every day who have that experience. They know they want more, but they don't know how to get it, even when simply taking a couple of steps will make the difference. It can mean catching yourself when you are behaving in a way that is not what you particularly want. It could be that you're gossiping or you're being negative about somebody.

All of those things make a big difference to who you are and what you represent. As we know, kefi is more than just a word describing a feeling: it encompasses the four pillars, the foundations of everything.

How do you bring more kindness into your life? Empathy and compassion start with yourself. Be kind to yourself. Treat yourself as your own best friend. Start thinking that you are good enough, that you can succeed. Do some small things: declutter your world, take yourself out, go for coffee. If you are desperately wanting a dress, save up for that dress. Avoid using your credit card, so you feel that you can afford to live fully in your life without constantly adding to your debt.

'Empower' means that you can achieve anything that you set your mind to. I've learnt that when I know that I can, then it means I can take a step in the right direction, and then another step. Before you know it, you'll be able to achieve that dream or goal that you've been looking to do.

It could be that you want to change jobs, because the people I talk to are often dissatisfied and unfulfilled in their jobs; being able to move into a job that is more fulfilling is something that many people aspire to. When you're passionate about what you do every day, life is much easier.

Freedom is being able to be 'you' without the stigma or the judgement of others. As Good Greek Girls, we've often lived with the shame, anxiety and anger that go with the judgement of not being good enough in the eyes of parents, siblings or other people. Luckily, this is becoming less and less common as the rest of us understand that it's not okay for our daughters, granddaughters and our nieces to be influenced by this sort of behaviour all the time.

Inspiration is enlightening; how do you live an inspired life when you take notice of your ideas? How do you work out the steps to achieve them? You're reading this book right now, this is the first port of call to be able to do that.

Many people tell me that it's hard to find your kefi – I used to think the same. In 2010, I went to Greece on a holiday with my mum and my two children, who were nine and thirteen at the time. I reconnected with my traditions, culture and heritage, while introducing it all to my children. They discovered a side to the family that they didn't know a lot about. The moment we landed back home, they were asking when we were going again. In 2017 I was able to revisit with my daughter – we had an amazing time with lots of laughs and kefi!

For a long time, I've been interested in how to improve myself and change things, but I wasn't sure quite how to get there. My desire to be a better person and to inspire others by passing it on has always been there.

After I left teaching in 2010 after my trip to Greece, I knew something had to change. I swanned around a little bit, not quite sure what to do next. I ended up doing some relief teaching, which I found to be fun and I became highly sought after. The following year, I attended a life coaching course and there I met some amazing people, including a very wonderful woman who became my best friend.

You've got to start catching when you are playing the comparison game: when you're saying, 'That stomach of mine is a bit big, my bum looks big in these jeans, I couldn't possibly be good enough to do that.' I often ran the program of, 'Who would love me? Why does it always have to happen to me? Nothing good ever happens, there's no good men out there,' and on and on and on. I was very good at having this negative self-talk.

I would also validate myself through stories of what other people had to say. My stories always said, 'Alex says that I am really good at doing that,' but nowhere did I represent my own point of view. During a life coaching session (the first I'd paid for, which was a huge turning point) I discovered that I was putting people on pedestals. I sought validation externally, from outside of me.

It wasn't until I was pulled up on the fact that I glorify other people's thoughts and I don't have any of my own that I actually realised what was going on. From that moment I could honestly say that things turned around for me in a huge way.

Quite a lot of people say to me, 'I don't know how to find my kefi.'

You can't just go and unpack the bags and think it's all going to happen automatically. It can be a slow process or a faster one, depending on what's going on for you. One small step is a giant leap for mankind, as we heard when Neil Armstrong stepped onto the moon, and it's a little bit like that with kefi.

We know what it looks like, we know what it feels like – but it's just out of our reach.

The first suggestion I have is to go through your Columns of Strength. Do an audit of your life and you'll find out what it is that you need to do.

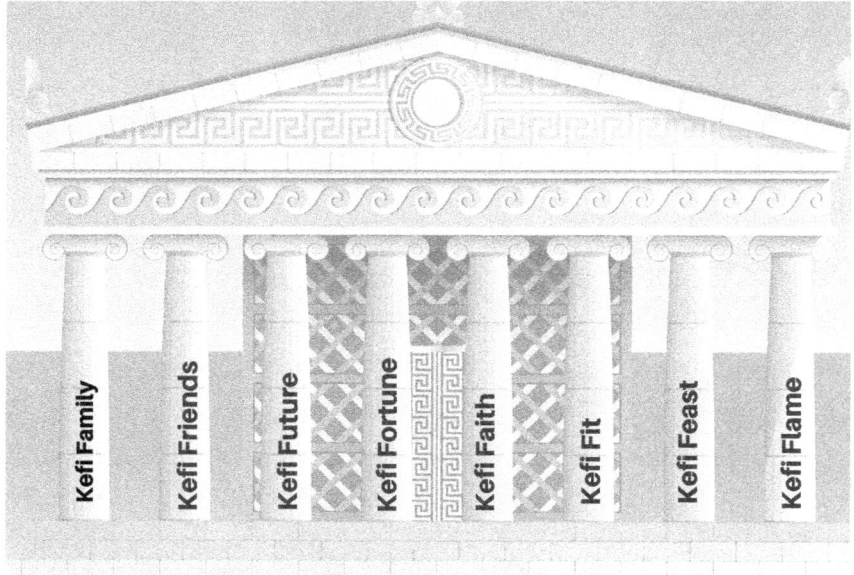

The Columns of Strength provide you with the ability to stand in your power, to cope with adversity that comes your way and to keep moving with a smile on your face. They give you the strength to stand firm in your convictions, beliefs and values no matter what. You get to value who you are, where you were and where you are now. With this strength you sail through life with grace, equanimity, and passion.

All of your stories and experiences contribute to the person you are today. These stories do not define who you are. More stuff will happen – you are now strong enough to do it all differently and be more.

There are eight Columns of Strength:

1) Kefi Family

2) Kefi Friends

3) Kefi Future

4) Kefi Fortune

5) Kefi Faith

6) Kefi Fit

7) Kefi Feast

8) Kefi Flame

Each of these will be discussed in this book.

The best thing about finding your kefi is that when things are going well, you feel light and happy and love life. There is no fighting or struggle involved in life. The real benefit of finding your kefi when times aren't at their best or times are tough in your daily life. When things are going well, everyone has their kefi, but what do you do when things aren't going so well?

Do you wake up in the morning with a spring in your step, ready for another day? Or do your drag yourself out of bed each day, dreading what is ahead? Have you got your kefi music cranked up loud? Are you dancing and having fun? Does the work you do bring you great joy and you feel as if it is not work at all? Or do you feel as if you are suffering every step of the way? Do you pick and choose where your kefi shows up in your life?

Getting clear on who you are and what you represent is important. Who do you want to work with? What have you got to offer? Every woman is a Kefi Chick and you determine how you live your own life your way. You have done your due diligence, you know who you are and what lights you up, you have got the power to be great! Honour your process and choose to do the tough stuff. Success needs you to focus on what you want in your business – doing the really important stuff, the non-negotiables.

Our busy lives play a role here. We beat ourselves up because we are so busy and there is no time for the important stuff in our lives.

For years I lived life in a blur, going through the motions. There was no kefi in my life. I could not see the joy. I felt lifeless and miserable, so I ate, disconnected from the important people in my life. I told myself I wasn't good enough; I blamed, I vented, I hated and so on. Step by step I evolved from that, as I found my kefi once more.

I gave myself permission to let go of a relationship which was not bringing out my potential. I reclaimed my extended family and friends, community and spirituality. I sold my house and released myself from the debt cycle. I changed career paths, starting up my business which is my passion. In the process, I discovered my sparkling jewel – my kefi!

As a teacher, it's quite easy for me to see how to teach someone to find things, but often the journey back to kefi means finding it yourself, uncovering the things that you like to do and experimenting a little bit.

Many people say to me, 'Oh, I can't do it on my own, it's just too hard – I don't know how to do it, I can't manage it, I'm just so alone.' There's often a lot of tears around this conversation.

What I suggest to you is this: make a commitment to book into a program and get some help with the process. Read this book to the end and do the work! Get the help that you need and take the outstretched hand that's being offered to you.

Many people say, 'I can't afford things.' Sometimes it's a case of making a decision, that you can afford something that's going to change the rest of your life. Perhaps it is possible to review your spending so you can put a little bit aside and save up for something that is important to you. There are things you can do which are free. Start with the suggestions at the end of each chapter which will assist you in increasing your kefi in your day to day life.

I often also hear, 'Nothing ever works for me.' What if this is the one thing that's going to make a difference? And what is the cost to you if you stay just as you are right now?

You can be the person who stays stuck or you can make the choice to change.

1)   Three action steps you can take to increase your kefi:

2) Complete an audit of your Columns of Strength. Look at each column and rate how things are working for you out of ten. Zero means absolutely nothing is working in any way shape or form. Ten means everything is perfect and there is no room for improvement. This will assist you to understand where you will take action to build capacity.

3) Self-date: take yourself out. Do something that you don't normally do: go somewhere new, do something fun and interesting. Take yourself out of your comfort zone. Maybe you would prefer something simpler and safer – run a bath, put some salts or a bath bomb in it, and light a candle. Create a romantic feeling for yourself. You're going to romance yourself and remind yourself that you are special.

4) Create tiny goals, select something you want to get done during the day. Write a list and pick the thing that is your top priority. Now break this task into 5–10 bite size pieces or steps. This helps you unpack what you need to do. The first step is simply to start. The idea is to make it simpler and to take out the thinking.

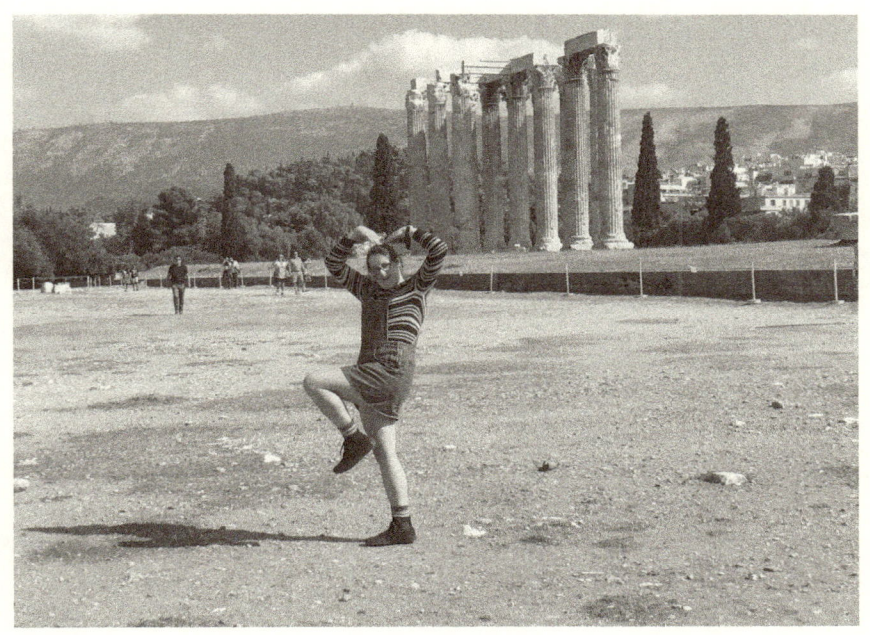

Chapter 3

Kefi Chick

'It's a terrible thing to go through life thinking that you have a rock on your side when you haven't.'
– Maria Callas, opera singer

'Be as you wish to be seen.'
– Socrates, philosopher

It is possible to spend your whole life attempting to prove to yourself and to others that you're good enough. Good Greek Girls 'people please', toe the line, avoid risk taking, repress their true feelings and attempt to get everything 'right'.

This is going to lead to resentment, anger and a lack of self-worth in the long run. Being a Good Greek Girl can play havoc on who you are, how you behave and what you do in life. The benefits of this are that you stay safe, do as you're told, never say no and behave in a perfect way.

Regardless of who you are, where you live, which part of Greece you are from, how old you are, what you do for work, whether you are married, divorced or single, run a business from your kitchen table, run a shop or have a full on enterprise, have children or not, are short, tall, slim, have love handles, can cook up a storm in the kitchen or can't boil an egg ...

There is a Good Greek Girl in you!

You know who she is! She rules the way you live your life. She shows you just what to do and how to do it. She keeps you safe from stepping outside the boundaries. You know there are several types of Good Greek Girls, because you are surrounded by them, and have grown up with them at family gatherings, at home and in the local community.

Each Good Greek Girl has a specific take on life. Does she give you the 'look' — you know, the one that lets you know exactly what she is thinking?

What are you wearing that for, it makes you look fat.

Look at her, she thinks she is something else.

You shouldn't say no.

What will people say?

You get the drift.

Being a Good Greek Girl can leave a successful and attractive woman struggling to find her ideal partner. It can leave a fabulous woman in a perpetual struggle with a particular member of her family. It can leave a strong intelligent woman stuck in an unfulfilling career.

For many women, being a Good Greek Girl means being stressed by family and teachers from a young age. It manifests itself in broken marriages, unfulfilled careers and parental challenges. There is an inability to receive any criticism without taking it personally.

There are many elements to being a Good Greek Girl; some are positive and serve you, others are negative and do not always serve you well. By finding out which sort of Good Greek Girl you are, you'll be able to work out how to stop being stuck as the person who doesn't always put themselves first.

Complete the online quiz here: <http://kefichicks.com/good-greek-girls-quiz/>.

So you have taken the quiz — what now? It's time to work out what you can do about it. You know that you don't want to end up perpetuating some of the things that you have seen from women in your family — women around you who have settled rather than stepping into their full potential.

Enjoy this moment and the next, regardless of what you are experiencing. As you cultivate the ability to find joy in the present, you call forward more reasons to be joyful. In every situation, you have opportunities to find blessings. Your happiness inspires others to transform their own sorrows into bliss. You can resolve your current question and situation by choosing the path of joy. What would bring more of it to your heart and soul?

There are five main types of Good Greek Girls, although there are others; maybe you are one type, or a bit of all of them.

The Rebel

You do all that you can to avoid family situations and are the opposite of what a Good Greek Girl 'should' be. You go out of your way to shun your inner Good Greek Girl and have no time for doing the right thing. You think it is all boring and not for you. You do as you please when you want, and think nothing of hurting other's feelings. You just want to block out the feelings you have when you are in the thick of it all – that way you don't have to really deal with anything or make meaningful connections.

The Perfectionist

As a Good Greek Girl you feel that every part of your life needs to be perfect – your children, your home, your appearance and how you behave. You are afraid that if something isn't perfect you will be judged, rejected, dismissed, or even ridiculed – so you drive yourself to constantly be more. At no time do you allow your high standards to slip. At times however, you become exhausted and slip into procrastination.

The People Pleaser

You are terrified no one will like you if you don't put everyone else first. You are into doing the 'right thing' like a Good Greek Girl is expected to do – it is only right to do this. You push yourself to make decisions based on how others will perceive you, so you over-give. You have few boundaries, as being seen as a good person is the most important thing for you. You have a need to be seen as a good person doing the right thing and keeping everyone happy. You are last on the list and you tell yourself that you can't put yourself first – what would people think?

The Overachiever

This is the Good Greek Girl doing it all. You crack the whip, always working on several things at once, doing everything to prove your value. You are addicted to the pursuit of goals, never questioning if you truly want the prize or result. You never pause to savour what you have achieved or completed, as you are already onto the next box to tick. Do you find it very difficult to relax, feeling guilty and unable to sit still for long? You tell yourself to get up and get on with it. You keep yourself so busy that you don't have time to feel things which make you uncomfortable.

The Comparison Queen

This Good Greek Girl is a '*ziliara*' or often jealous, looking to see what everyone has and is doing. When you have created something really special – a cake, a new business idea, a gorgeous new outfit, shoes, bag – she pops up and flaunts someone else's stuff in your face. You might say, 'I suppose that is nice, but have you seen this?' You remind yourself that you don't really measure up to your standards; you feel crappy about yourself and not good enough. You fall into a heap quickly when this happens, as you tell yourself you will never catch up to those other people.

Some of the common things Good Greek Girls do include the following.

- She tells herself the same stories in her head to justify the way she behaves.

- She is unforgiving.

- She repeats herself and can have a conversation in her head that she would never have with anyone in person.

- She often mirrors people such as a critical parent, grandparent, aunt or teacher.

- She self-sabotages and stops being herself.

It's good to realise that you can't control how others view you, and you can't make them like you. No matter how hard you try, it isn't going to assist you to become the person that you wish to be.

Get over that one and be yourself.

Good Greek Girls are usually people pleasers. And they always do what someone else wants them to do. Well, here's a tip. It's time to slow down and get out of the auto pilot of doing what everybody else wants. Take the time to ask yourself what you would like to do first. Then get started on it. Before you know it, you're going to be in a great space.

Being Good Greek Girls, we spend a lot of time growing up, being what we think we should be – or the antithesis of it, as we fight to become the person we think we should be. That's where we often see rebels coming out through the family – the ones who say no all the time and are forever fighting as opposed to the meek, mild 'yes' person who can't fight the family.

Often, we can't see the great life out there that is available to us. We immerse in martyrdom and expect others to read our minds. We love moaning about how we do so much for others and yet no one understands and sees us. You feel invisible and you just don't know what to do with yourself.

Traditionally speaking, Good Greek Girls don't rock the boat. They don't backchat to their parents, they don't smoke in front of their parents – at least, they didn't in the past. They don't move out on their own, they don't live with their boyfriend before they get married, they don't have sex before marriage and they never say no. They do as they're told and follow the rules.

Imagine how wonderful it will be when you honour your truth and share what you think, instead of being ruled by this group of unwritten rules and laws and ways of behaviour that somebody, somewhere, thought were important.

Trusting the process and trusting in a long term resolution that's in your best interest is going to assist you to evolve even further.

The most amazing thing of all, however, is that you're going to find your voice. I know that when I was younger, I was such a people pleaser. I found it exceptionally difficult to say what I wanted to say and to get my needs met. I couldn't say no, I just didn't know how. I would take care of others — at least I thought I was. I felt exhausted all the time and I felt tired.

My voice sounded like I had a permanent fishbone stuck in my throat. All I wanted was approval and validation. I just wanted to be liked. I wanted to avoid disapproval at any cost — so much so that during friendships, I wouldn't actually say the truth. I would allow people to walk all over me and to say things that probably weren't very kind or nice.

I can remember being fifteen or sixteen, when I really hated gossip. I still do, but I really hated it back then and I was very clear about not participating in it. In later years, you get dragged into it and I wasn't so stoic and regimented in holding on tight to my value.

What I know for sure is that the Good Greek Girl role is going to rob you of your life, particularly if you're looking at the parts of it that are holding you back, that define your identity in ways that are *not* you.

Being a Good Greek Girl is not always negative; it can be very empowering and enlightening. It can provide you with a sense of knowing who you are, when you are doing the things that you wish to do for you. It's focusing on the 'good girl' component that stops you being who you're meant to be — that's the part we're focusing on, rather than the negative components.

For a long time, I was always second in charge of things. Many times over I would be second in command or vice president or the helper or the 'secretary'; I would be assisting the person who was in charge, the head teacher or the president of a community committee I was on, or the chairperson. I found that I was over-giving, because I wanted everything to be right and I wanted everything to succeed. However, I was actually giving up what I needed for me.

I was working really hard, running myself ragged and doing their work for them, because I was loving it – but I also wanted to be validated by what I was doing. I just wanted to be seen.

I helped them look good and did the background work as the consummate helper. I found that this happened in quite a number of other areas in my life as well, such as friendships or when I was exploring spiritual practices – and that's not a great place to be in.

I get asked if the art of self-care is arrogant and selfish. I believe that you must look after yourself. If you let yourself go – as I know I have when going to the pantry, eating myself silly and wondering why I was putting on weight overnight – then you need to correct this.

Look after yourself and your body, eat nourishing food and invest in yourself. Whether you can do it on your own or with a friend, or whether you need some professional assistance, there are some amazing life coaches out there at the moment.

No matter what you do, if you invest in *you* then you're going to be showing your daughters, sons, nieces, nephews and the children around you how important it is to take care of yourself.

My main mission is to make sure that the young people coming after us don't have to go through the same experiences as generations of women – Greek, Italian, Polish, Australian, all walks of life – which have been held back.

I want people to move forward and to make sure that this crazy, guilt-ridden 'holding us back' syndrome is able to be cleared and healed, so that the girls going forward know that they can have what they need to have, with respect to the women who have gone before us.

What do I do now? What are some of the things I used to think were selfish? I exercise every day for 60 minutes. Rain, hail or shine. I used to think I couldn't go walking in the rain and the cold, but I have discovered that it's actually quite enjoyable. I eat nourishing food by choice and have stopped medicating my emotions with sweets, chocolate, bread, cake, biscuits, chips, etc. I take time out – sometimes I don't answer the phone. I spend time on my deck of an evening, enjoying my view on my own.

I know that if I feel tired, I need to stop. I had some health issues a couple of years ago, and I had a hysterectomy which made me stop and take stock.

I surround myself with people who are smart, self-aware and only interested in two-way relationships. For so long I was in one-way relationships.

I eliminated the clutter, creating a soul-nourishing workspace. My home environment is very different; every day I get my finances in order and I never make choices to buy or not buy things out of guilt or obligation.

Finding your ability to say 'no' so that you don't feel conflicted and guilty is challenging for a lot of people, but it can be possible. The first step is to actually notice that you are saying yes when you actually meant to say no.

What do you do when you don't feel good enough? I know that I hear quite often and I've said it myself, 'Nothing I do is every good enough for my mother/father/sister/brother/grandparents ... nothing I do is ever good enough for my husband, my son, my daughter.' It goes on as a learned pattern that you've picked up.

By whose standards are you making these decisions? By whose standards are you saying that you're not good enough?

Think of three things that you are good at and take notice, because you are worthy. I see you, others see you and we acknowledge you. Do you have trouble showing your true emotions or judging yourself by someone else's standards?

Your true emotions are really important. As we know, Good Greek Girls don't get angry or cry, Good Greek Girls don't laugh at the wrong moment, Good Greek Girls aren't loud, blah blah blah.

Some tips to avoid reverting to being a Good Greek Girl who is not being her authentic self:

- Realise you cannot control how other people view you or make them like you.

- Slow down and get out of the auto pilot of pleasing.

- Honour your truth and share what you think.

- Forget perfectionism.

- Don't be afraid to be different.

- Be true to yourself.

- Remember you are worthy, you are good enough!

- Feel your true emotions.

- Release the pain.

- Be defined by self-acceptance and confidence.

- Build your self-esteem.

- Surround yourself with people who build you up rather than tear you down.

- Say no when you want to and say yes when you want to.

- Remember – life starts with YOU!

Three action steps you can take to increase your kefi:

1) Journal what you think a Good Greek Girl is. Ask yourself where she shows up in my life and how you feel about it. Allow yourself to explore the process.

2) Complete the Good Greek Girl quiz that is available online and the link is here: <http://kefichicks.com/good-greek-girls-quiz/>. Discover which Good Greek Girl is most dominant.

3) Observe when you say yes instead of saying no and then you are conflicted. Awareness is key – that's the first port of call. Review how you say it as well. Do you speak

with good grace or with resentment? First step is to see it happen; the next is to increase awareness as soon as possible, then to catch yourself and change how you do this. Even if you change your mind and say so is doable.

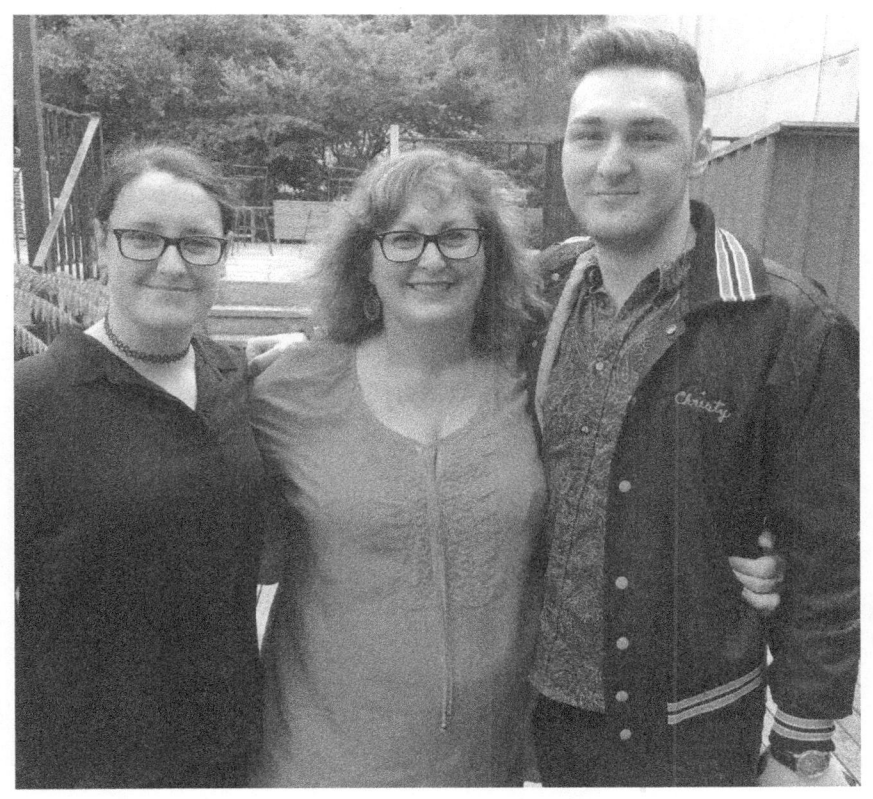

Chapter 4

Kefi Family

'What you leave behind is not what is engraved in stone monuments, but what is woven into the lives of others.'
— **Pericles, general**

The relationship between Greek daughters and their mothers can be one of the most challenging, demanding and confrontational relationships on the one hand — and on the flipside, it can be liberating, loving and unconditional. The love between a mother and daughter is an interesting field. In some cases, mother and daughter are so alike that they end up feeling that they're clashing all the time, rather than valuing their likenesses. They only see the differences.

Having the unconditional love of your mother is something that every person in every culture everywhere needs. When you have unconditional love, you know that you can achieve anything. It does not mean, however, that you manipulate or control that love in a situation to get the things done your way.

How wonderful is it to be able to be happy in each other's company? To be happy with your mum and your dad and other members of your family? A Kefi Family is one where everyone enjoys and embraces each other, regardless of difference of values or beliefs. There is communication, loud talking and laughter — you know where to go when you need support or a helping hand.

A Kefi Family is one that shows love no matter what. A Kefi Family will be there for you when times are tough and when times are great. Your Kefi Family can sometimes be quite challenging, because they can also criticise, judge and bring out the worst in you, or at least that's what you think.

It is wonderful to be able to enjoy your family when you all get together. My mother is one of six brothers and sisters. The husbands, wives, first cousins and our grandparents would all gather around the table. There would be the adults table and a separate kids table where we got to hang out with our cousins. The table would always be groaning with an abundance of food: there was always spanakopita made by *yiayia* (grandmother), *psari* (fish) mayonaisa as a family favourite, crayfish and other seafood (back when it was more affordable). We enjoyed many lively conversations, some with tears but mostly with laughter. To this day, when the opportunity arises for the family to get together even in much smaller groups these days, there is always food involved.

Christmas with family is always a blessing with food, a crowd of people and lots of loud talking. My mother's favourite saying was, 'It's hard to be a member of this family,' always with a great big smile on her face. She loved saying this to any new partners on their first family experience. So what exactly was going on with the family get-togethers? Lots of love, and loads of kefi!

Enjoying your family is the most important component. Overlooking the parts that you don't like so much can be tough, especially when a Greek family is involved. Good Greek Girls can be challenged when surrounded by extended family. Words get sucked in and held inside the body. Then there's the pain of the hurtful words you hear from the uncle or aunt who have nothing nice to say. Things like, 'You look fat today, you will never get a husband looking like that,' or, 'When are you getting engaged/married, having children, buying a house, getting a job?' and so on. You take the painful comment and stuff it in, then add some of the delicious food you are surrounded with, and it holds it all nicely in place inside your body.

You don't want to end up resentful, sick, stressed, angry or disconnected, because that is the absolute truth. If you only find the negative when it comes to your family, you forget to embrace the whole. You'll find that you will be on the outer rim and you'll feel alone and stressed, and not connected with the family. Many clients say to me things like, 'My sisters just don't get me — they don't see that I am alone on the weekend. They are busy and never think to invite me.' Or, 'My mother or father constantly pick on me, nothing is ever good enough for them.' I hear these stories on a regular basis. I usually ask if they think that their parents are doing the best job that they can with the resources available. The answer is always yes.

The first Column of Strength is Kefi Family. Make no mistake: without family, you will find it exceptionally challenging to do the things that you wish to do. Your family is your rock, your base, your connection, your foundation. They are the people who will assist you when times are tough or when times are exciting and joyous.

When you are embraced by your Kefi Family, you can be who you truly are. You don't get shut down; you don't feel that you're not enough, that you're unworthy of being part of the family, because everybody criticises and shuts you down. In actual fact, people say these things because they are your family and they love you; they want to see you achieving more, especially when you are underachieving.

Quite often you'll find that the things that you think are part of the negative brigade are the parts that are challenging you. They're doing it for your own good — it just doesn't feel like it at the time. When you're not in a good place, any criticism or suggestion can feel like you are being yelled at. A Kefi Family welcomes each other into their homes and has connected conversations; there is support between one another. You can make mistakes and feel safe and accepted. It's fun being part of this type of family. It's enjoyable. It's something that you look forward to.

I'm one of seventeen first cousins and when we get together, we often have so much fun. One time we were sitting around a fire; one of my aunts was living on a farm at the time and the female cousins present were sitting outside in a circle around this fire pot. We had cousins who had come from interstate and it had been a while since we'd been together. One cousin said the fateful words, 'Well, what's news?'

Another cousin said, 'Well, I've just separated from my boyfriend.'

A third said, 'Yes I've just done that too.'

It was my turn: 'I've decided to separate from my husband today.'

There was raucous laughter afterwards, because no one had expected that the simple words 'what's news' would have such a dramatic effect. To this day we often remind ourselves and reminisce about how hilarious it was, when a simple statement procured so much news.

The shocking truth is that there's lots of things between mothers, daughters and sisters: clashing, potential angst and anxiety, when all the other is doing is saying things out of love, to make you a better person.

I know this to be true because I've experienced it first hand. Not very long ago, I made a monumental decision.

I had no money to pay my mortgage and it was the end of the school holidays and I didn't have any teaching work, because the schools were closed and I was using my credit cards until that point. The problem was, my credit cards were maxed out; I was short of money and I wasn't going to make it through to the end of the school holidays before work started again.

I had to do something new. My finances weren't going all that well and I got some financial advice.

When I went to see this person, with great pain in his voice he said to me, 'Irini, you need to sell your house, pay off all your debts and move in with your mother.'

That's exactly what I did. It turned my life around.

My mother was a lady of great character, strength and determination. She had been chair of a Greek festival near where we live, which is coming up for its twenty-fifth year. She was heavily involved in the Greek community and she gave to many charities. She was a go getter; if you wanted something done, you asked my mother. What I discovered when I moved in with my mum was that we had lots of shared activities that we enjoyed doing; before I knew it, they called me by my mother's name, number two. I was attempting to follow in her footsteps.

It is just over a year since she passed away at the time of writing this, and I find I am continuing her legacy in giving to the local Greek community.

The challenge is, when you are someone who is capable and able to get things done, you often end up being someone that people want to do all the jobs. What I learnt was that it's okay to do some of the things that I could see my mum involved in, because that was how I celebrated our connection. This is how I connected with our traditions, culture and heritage. This is how I gained my identity: by being part of the things that were important to my family. Learning to step back when required has been a huge lesson and using that little two letter word – 'no' – is so powerful. I learnt it is okay to say no, the sky won't fall down and people won't like you less!

My family came to Australia in the early 1900s and they were one of the first Greek families to settle in Hobart. They gave so much to their community, both the Australian and the Greek. Living with my mother, I learnt to celebrate the good things and understand what it is to change – and that I don't have to do everything the way that it was done in the past. There was no need to be over-responsible and to carry the burden of the family legacy.

This also allowed me to develop my self-awareness. One of the main keys in this Column of Strength, Kefi Family, is to understand that you can catch yourself to stop over-reacting or over-giving when you're with loved ones. The only person you can actually change is yourself.

Family is important. Family includes your children, parents, cousins – and as we know, in a Greek family we value our extended family very deeply. We are a village in our own right.

Understanding and retaining that connection keeps the story alive for the family. Christmas was once a happy time and over the years we've found that because we've married and had children and the family has grown, having the big extended family Christmas became much more challenging. There is a part of the family that is really looking forward to instigating this again this year. As our parents are leaving us, we find that we are becoming closer again, starting our own traditions for the next generations.

Accepting that you have a lot of similarities with your parents and grandparents will build your identity. Acceptance comes from embracing the whole of a person, and ultimately finding happiness and peace in their presence is paramount.

I often work with clients who find it challenging to be around their family. They talk about their sisters or parents being an issue, and they find it hard to be the person that they need to be. When you are comfortable with yourself, you can step in and out of your family situation much more easily. Taking everything they say to heart is going to be detrimental to you in the long run. Instead, be strong and to listen to your inner compass.

All families challenge you – that's the point. They're supposed to help you grow and bring out your potential. The moment that you decide that it can be different, you're going to find that it's going to be easy, and you'll be able to strengthen and enhance those relationships.

You can turn your relationships around. Start by making contact. Call your sister every day. Call your mother every day. Have a short conversation. Let them know that you care, because often what you're doing is pushing them away. Bring them closer to you and you'll find your relationship will develop.

I also hear, 'My family always criticises and judges me.' This may be true; have a look and see if there's truth to any of the story. Perhaps there's something that you're not doing and that you're in denial about. Journaling can help with this process.

Sometimes it's not about you at all; what they're seeing is themselves in you. They don't want someone else to make the same mistakes that they did – this observation can be important.

I also hear, 'Nothing is ever good enough for my mother/stepmother/daughter/etc.' Remember your mother is doing the best job that she can with the resources that she's got — that is, all the things that she knows how to do. Generational imprinting is also at play here; maybe she's repeating what she got told as a young woman as well. Think about that. Understand where what she's saying has come from.

I have extremely fond memories of the Hobart Botanical Gardens as a child, because Mum would give up her afternoon off from the shop to do activities with us kids which we would enjoy, rather than what she would enjoy. The strongest memory I have is of the flower clock, which is covered in flowers in spring and early summer. My sister, my brother and I would run around playing chasey, while Mum would sit and relax away from the daily grind of the 'bloody' shop.

I remember the day that Mum found out Dad was dying — I just didn't know what the news was. He couldn't bear to tell her himself, so the doctor broke the news to her. I, like any thirteen year old, was immersed in my own teenage self so had no idea why Mum yelled at me to stop trying to ring the radio station and win a prize (most likely the album of the day). I found out later that the doctor had told him, 'You have six weeks to live, get your affairs in order.' He was so shocked that he couldn't verbalise what the doctor told him. Life changed that day. Dad was in and out of hospital; the smell of hospital disinfectant still takes me back to visiting him.

Mum and Dad had bought a house not far from where we lived in the shop. One day we were living upstairs in the shop, the next day Mum and her sister had moved us into our new home. Dad lived a further two weeks after our move. We kids had not been told anything about what was wrong with Dad. One night my sister asked what we dreaded to ask. 'Cancer,' Mum said, 'your dad has cancer.' Okay, that is not good, but people take a while to die from that don't they? It turns out they can die quickly too! I believe Dad lost the will to live once he had been told the news.

How do you process that news when you are thirteen years old? Being a Good Greek Girl I heard all sorts of things, like, 'He doesn't want anyone crying and carrying on over his coffin,' which I thought meant he didn't want anyone to cry. I kept hearing Mum say we need to be strong; I guessed that meant you couldn't cry. I heard other people say, 'Be strong, stand tall and remember your dad.' How do you grieve the main man of your life?

I have to say that I didn't do relationships well with men in my life. I didn't know to be friends, how to trust and how to be me.

For so many years I struggled to say what I wanted to say. I said what I thought I should say, what others wanted me to say. I was out of touch with my own needs and wants. That has changed; now I am more articulate in voicing my wants and needs. Understanding my family values has had a huge impact on become a Kefi Chick.

Three action step you can take as a result of reading Kefi Family to help you become stronger:

1) Reflection: what is important for you and your family? How do you want your family members to interact with each other? What values are important for your family? Take some time to think about this to consider what is working or what is not.

2) Imagine life's a stage. Draw a circle stage like you see in Ancient Greece such as Herodotus' Theatre or at Epidaurus, and put yourself in the middle. List the members in your family. Think about where your family members fit around you in stage: who's closest and who's furthest away, and who would you like to bring closer. Awareness of where you place your family members will assist you in operating your own family.

3) Do something special your family likes to do. This can be something you like to do with your mother or grandmother. It could be spending some time cooking or sewing. Perhaps you're going to host a get-together. Make it about the whole family. There are so many things that you can do to bring your family together.

Remember, family is important and you're part of a whole.

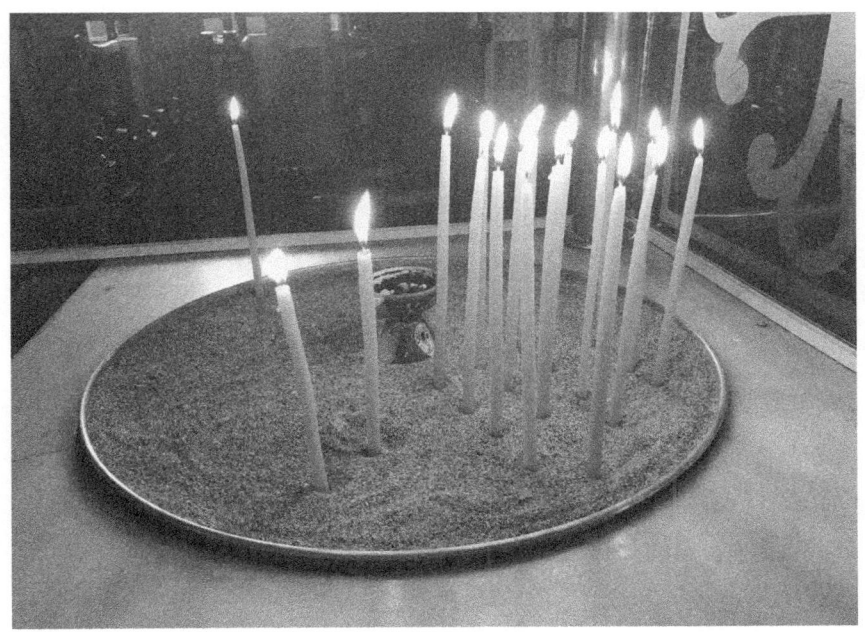

Chapter 5

Kefi Friends

'I don't need a friend who changes when I change and who nods when I nod; my shadow does that much better.'
— Plutarch, general

'My best friend is the man who in wishing me well, wishes it for my sake.'
— Aristotle, philosopher

Friends can be our biggest teachers, cheer squad and supporters. At other times they can be toxic, treacherous and daunting. True friends, they say, you can count on one hand. Some of us have been lucky enough to share love as a friendship. That person who you get on with, the person who gets you.

There may be other times in your life when you feel as you are a ghost: you're invisible, no one cares for you and you're totally alone. It can be a tough when you feel abandoned and deserted.

The truth is, being your own best friend is where it all starts. How do you treat yourself? How do you talk to yourself? How's your mindset towards yourself? Do you love and support *you* first? Or do you beat yourself up and tell yourself that you're not good at anything?

The first port of call when it comes to friendship is when a true friend loves you unconditionally and is there for you through thick and thin, sharing your experiences.

Maybe it's that person who you call you just want to tell them about that guy who likes you or how your mother's driving you crazy. Maybe you want to share that your career is in pieces or you hate your job: 'What should I do?' That person who's such a good friend that you can tell them anything, even the things that you know keeping locked inside of you will have a toxic effect.

Friends trigger our empathy, compassion and trust. Friends love you; Kefi Friends love you just as you are. They support you when times are tough; they stick around and hold the space for you when you need them to. They check in and ask if you're okay. They allow you to be free and to be you.

Kefi friendships feed and nurture you; they are light and airy rather than heavy and draining. You love being with each other.

Sometimes people are lucky enough to have a circle of friends who fit the bill; other times, some people feel that they have no one at all to share their lives with on a friendship level. And it's what you do when you have no one that can make a huge impact on you. What do you do? Sometimes it's about reaching out and making a phone call to someone you haven't seen in a while, reconnecting in that way.

A Kefi Friend is someone you can trust with your secrets. A Kefi Friend is someone who you can have fun together with. That really hearty, belly aching laugh, the one that really feels like you've let off some steam. Hanging out with people who get you and make you feel safe is something that is very special. It is your circle of trust that buoys you, keeps you afloat, nourishes you.

At all costs you need to enjoy these friendships and they need to be reciprocal – you need to avoid frenemies. A frenemy is someone who pretends that they're a friend, but at the same time they're trying to beat you down and undo all the things that you're doing. They aren't the true person who keeps you sane. They're not the person who keeps your secrets, because they go out spreading them behind your back.

Some people think that a frenemy is better than no friend at all. But what is this 'friendship' costing you?

Oh, you should hear what she had to say about you to her

other friends. Off they go in a tirade, sharing all your secrets and then creating trouble behind your back. They want to feel significant and superior to you. They want you to be lower than them in the pecking order so they feel better about themselves.

I work with several clients who have difficulty sorting their friendships. They're so desperate to have friends that they let down their filters for what they'll accept from a friend. Sometimes a friend in a relationship is surrounded by single friends who attempt to sabotage the relationship and create a flurry of rumour and innuendo. They are happiest when the friend in the relationship is having issues and comes crying to them.

Communication is key when it comes to friendship. You need someone who really listens – someone who understands your core needs and meets them. Someone who is certain to be your friend through thick and thin. This person makes you feel significant and loves you unconditionally, helping you grow and bring out your potential.

There are times when a friendship is not what it appears to be. According to a recent UK study, differing opinions, lifestyles and senses of humour mean 45% of people have frenemies in their friendship circle[1]. Some friends aren't even liked, but it's considered easier to keep them as a 'friend'. How can this be a reality? For what reason is the friendship circle compromised because of this enemy in their midst?

This can end up with you feeling stressed, angry, disconnected and alone while surrounded by an unproductive circle of

---

1   Francis, G 2017, 'Frenemies: Shocking research reveals millions of Brits "can't stand" their own friends', *The Sun*, <https://www.thesun.co.uk/living/4036891/brits-dont-like-friends-survey/>.

friends. There's lots of judgement around those relationships. Who wants to be sitting at home, staring at the walls, feeling jealous with nowhere to go? Would you really rather hang out with that controlling friend who gets you to do things you don't want to do?

What's the point of feeling resentful, frustrated or drained when you're around people who don't bring out the best in you – who aren't looking out for you as their number one priority as a friend?

Understanding who and what you believe as friendship is something very important. Over time I've had some friends who have been drainers. Some people call them energy vampires. Sometimes I thought I was helping them; in reality they just did what they wanted anyway.

Have you ever felt you were drifting away from a friend, but didn't know what to do? It's easier to break up with a boyfriend than it is with a controlling friend. They control where you go, what you wear, what you eat, who you're married to, who you go out with – all that sort of thing. Sometimes you end up as a passive participant in the relationship as you self-preserve and keep yourself safe. It is just easier in the long run.

You can also get the people who are so sad that all they want to do is tell you their sad story over and over and over again, like a broken record. They stay in a dark spiral, validated by telling you their tale of woe. This then becomes an anchor and they connect to you in this way every time they see you. It's like press the play button for sadness every time.

You need to reflect on what is happening around you so that you value yourself. You'll have the best possible relationships by positioning yourself as a good friend and setting clear boundaries. If you have needy friends, you've got to keep them out of your inner circle. Friendship is at its best when you are your best self with the people around you.

There have been times in my life when I've had a series of needy friends, who have tried to monopolise my time, wanted my emotional energy and support.

I've found that I kept them in my life because they made me feel safe and significant. One time I observed this was when I had recently separated from my husband of twelve years. I had moved into a new home and I had some people, at least three at a time, who would ring me on a regular basis for advice. Or they would want some support from me at a time when I needed to support my children and remain focused on my own personal healing journey. I found that this proved to be a huge distraction for a number of years.

During my personal development journey, I made a very close friend with somebody; it was almost like we had our friendship on speed. We spoke every day about all sorts of things. This person was exciting and energetic, and we got on like a house on fire.

Somewhere along the line, something changed for both of us. Sometimes I've had experiences where friends just walk out of my life without a reason. Or they walk out because it seemed to be the right time for them and I was quite a bit uncertain. It was one of the things that triggered abandonment in my mind and I started having feelings about my own lack of worthiness.

As I learnt to become more self-aware, I was able to observe which relationships were best for me in the long run. When I was at primary school I had a few mean girls making fun of me.

I learnt to be silent; to avoid conflict at all costs and not speak my mind. I learnt to say what I thought people wanted to hear.

There was one girl in particular who was quite mean. Every time I was around her I wouldn't say anything, so I wouldn't be picked on.

When I was around the age of fourteen I met a boy, and of course Good Greek Girls do not have boyfriends when they're fourteen. Good Greek Girls do not go to the movies and hold hands with a boy.

I also learnt was how cruel and two-faced people could be. One of my so-called friends at the time had a birthday party and they invited the full circle of friends except for me, because for some reason their father had decided that I was a bad influence.

I'm not quite sure why he thought that, but sometimes people say things without thinking about why they're saying them, especially when you're a teenager.

I wasn't invited to the party and it was heartbreaking, because our families had been friends for a very long time and it wasn't really obvious why that was happening. But I did learn that they were no longer my friends — that was a certainty. I became clearer about who I should hang out with at school.

What I did learn is that sometimes you have to suck it up, because I had to go to the party and get two of my other friends, because we were going to a Greek dancing festival to a performance. It was very embarrassing that I had to knock on the door and ask for the girls to come out.

It was something that has stayed with me for many, many

years. Sometimes things happen when we're young and we don't understand why, but before we know it it's turned into a monumental issue. Interestingly, these people probably had no idea how that affected me for a long time after.

When you have your kefi, you attract the right friends, the people who lift you up. You attract the people who are a perfect match, just like when you're looking to attract a partner into your life.

I have a friend who has experienced a lot of adversity in her life. We often talk about our friends and how some friends take advantage of us because of her kind nature. They think they're entitled to it for whatever reason.

My friend says it's useful to listen to your internal antenna, because that's how you know when someone is right for you. If you've met someone and you have feelings, you can feel your stomach churning, that's probably a sign that you should be paying attention. If you first meet someone and you feel a bit drained, that's a sign that you should be paying attention.

A lot of people say to me that it's really hard to find good friends these days and that any friend is a good friend. In response I say to please evaluate how they make you feel when you are with them.

Is any friend a good friend if they're using and abusing you? Perhaps they're coming around and eating out of your fridge every day? Or they're dropping off their children before they go off and do stuff, because you're the nice one and you just want to be liked and validated by someone else? But perhaps the shoe doesn't fit, because when it comes to your turn, somehow they're always busy and you can't leave your children with them?

Finding new friends can be quite challenging. Sometimes you could meet new people through other friends; you might invite someone to bring a friend along for coffee. I remember meeting two lovely ladies at church – I call them my church friends. A few years ago, one day we were just talking and somewhere along the line we said we'll go for coffee. So, we did. It has now every Sunday after church for the three of us. Sometimes a couple of other people join us, but we've created a friendship of like-minded people who are there to support each other, and it's actually really interesting and liberating. This friendship began from a conversation and a realisation of things in common.

Other people tell me that you just can't trust anyone anymore. Having trust issues means you don't trust yourself to be able to discern who is a potential good friend. But it takes trial and error. Sometimes you make a friend and you think, 'Oh, they're not showing me their true self.' That is okay. Give it a go and see what comes of it.

Other people only have friends on Facebook, where they message each other and like posts, showing friendship that way. So often now we see people who are dreading going onto Facebook to see that people haven't liked their post or are making negative comments.

The thing is, having friends in real life encourages you to have good habits and it can chase away depression and dissatisfaction issues. It helps you feel satisfied and happy. Ultimately, as we know, we're looking for happiness and because we are people who require social connection, having people around us who love and appreciate us is the number one priority.

Kefi Friends are where it's at. It's a core issue for us and knowing who you love and appreciate.

The other side of this coin is that you need to be able to *be* the friend that you wished to have. Maybe you are reaching out and making phone calls, taking a risk to get to know someone new. I know some people who say, 'I'm the only one who ever rings up.' You need to be aware of this to be able to break the cycle; this is how to encourage and nurture a new friendship, or to keep the lines of communication open with your current friends.

Three action steps you can take as a result of reading Kefi Friends:

1) List five top qualities of good friends. What do you need from your friends that you reciprocate? Think about the things that you value too, so that you are a match for the people who are in your life as friends.

2) Journaling is a great way to work out how you feel about your friendships. Think about your circle of friends – who is in your inner circle, those trusted friends who you share your heart with? Do you need to move on from any of your friends? Do you need to break up from any frenemies, the people who you find are challenging?

3) Go out on a 'Kefi Friends' date. Do something fun together: maybe go to a Greek dance or fitness class, go for coffee, go to the movies, go to a day spa, go for a walk – there

are so many options. Visit each other with your children and have them play together so that you can have some girl time. Spending quality time with friends is important.

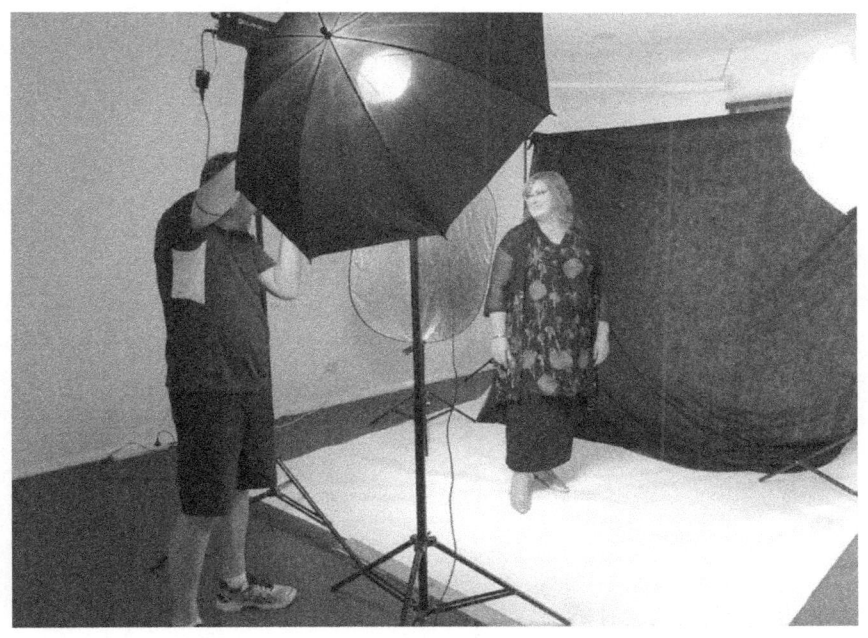

Chapter 6

Kefi Future

'Pleasure in the job puts perfection in the work.'
— **Aristotle, philosopher**

'Success is dependent on effort.'
— **Sophocles, playwright**

It can be a challenge to know what you want to do with your life when you are an adult, let alone when you are a young person with so many options to choose from. Some future jobs haven't even been created for our children today. So much confusion and uncertainty can contribute to a lack of direction in life. Years ago you chose your profession and you stuck to it for life, no matter what. Now it's not so simple; it's common for people to change jobs every five years, or even less for some, as they search for meaning and connection with a job that they find fulfilling.

From a young age, individuals are asked, 'What career path will you take? What are your dreams? Where will you be in five, ten or twenty years?' So often I hear, 'I have no idea what I want to do, I am not good at anything, I can't decide.' Many Greek parents, and many other migrants, want their kids to be lawyers and doctors in particular as they are good solid, stable, respectful professions. They are certain that this will result in a happy and wealthy life, avoiding the poverty and hardship they experienced before coming to Australia.

I can remember growing up as a young Good Greek Girl, hearing about the sort of professions that were desirable. I went to a girls' school and in those days the main professions were teaching and nursing. I chose primary school teaching – 'a great profession for a woman' is what I heard. 'You can take care of your children in the holidays and you have good hours.' I remember being at university sitting around the 'wog table' talking about our career paths and how we wanted to please our parents. We would laugh and joke about what would happen if we didn't pass, which did happen for some people — they ended up just fine, doing something that they wanted to do.

Looking at your future includes looking at your career and where you want to be in a few years' time — looking at the dreams that you have for yourself and perhaps your family, working out how to achieve them. When you don't know what you want for yourself, life can be confusing and uncertain. Having a Kefi Future, where you do all that you possibly can to live the life you dream of, will contribute to your happiness. It means having clarity, understanding the steps to get there and, most important of all, knowing *why*!

Often, people feel that they don't have dreams. They have no idea what they want as other things are preventing clarity of thought. Do you live day to day, week to week, month to month? Do you 'go with the flow' and wait for opportunity to come to you like a lottery prize?

Dreams are the things that you aspire to — the things that you look forward to and hope will happen. On the opposite side, when you have no dreams, you feel static and like there's absolutely no movement whatsoever. Knowing what your desires are, what you'd like for your future, helps you work out what you want to achieve.

And then you can work out the steps that you need to take to succeed.

If you know that you want to go on a holiday, you know what the steps are: you need to work out the financing, tickets, destinations, who you're going with, a passport (if needed), accommodation, booking tours and other things like that.

Before you start this process, the very first thing is to make the decision that you will go on a holiday, as the other steps follow on from making the decision. Sometimes this decision is the hard part, so looking at the decision-making process is part of the whole segment of Kefi Future. When you make decisions, there are several things you can assess.

- Is the decision good for me?

- Will it impact on anyone else?

- What do I need to know?

- Do I have enough information?

- What are the positives?

- What are the negatives?

How wonderful is it when you have career fulfilment? When you are working in an area where you're passionate, energetic, fulfilled and love being there? When getting out of bed in the morning is easy and there's a spring in your step?

Having the best career for you is going to make sure that you are fulfilled. You're also showing the children around you what it looks like to enjoy work rather than seeing work as drudgery. There is nothing worse than seeing someone dragging themselves out of bed every day to head off to a soul-destroying job.

Looking at how you want your family connection to be in the future is also part of this story. Your Kefi Future is one where you're feeling happy. Look into the future: how are you going to feel? What are you going to see and hear? How are you going to think about what's going on around you? It is all about how you will feel in the future with your family, which is filled with kindness and empowerment.

In your future, do you see your home as your castle? How does your home look? After I separated and left the family home that we had built together, I had quite a rebuilding process ahead of me. I had moved away from my family early on when we built a lovely home by a river. This was new and challenging for me in so many ways. After I moved back to the city, I was able to purchase my own home and had to reassess where I was heading. I saw that as a 'stepping stone' home; it was not the home that I really wanted, but it was certainly the home that would give me shelter and safety for the next few years, as well as providing my children a place close to their school.

Fast forward, I now live in pretty much my dream home. It's newly built and has enough space for myself and my daughter. It has a view of the water and the mountain, which is something I always wanted. It is fresh and clean and new. I call it my hotel house. It is easy to maintain and keep clean; here I feel at peace and happy.

Is your home your castle? Is your home the place where you feel at peace, where you know that your kefi can be restored? Is it a place where you feel you're at home? If you've said no to any of those questions, I suggest you have a look at what you can do to change things. Perhaps it's to do with the clutter, the styling of your home, or with how you make it look.

Another part of your Kefi Future is lifestyle. Are you living the way that you always thought you would? I'm not talking out of control stuff like being rich and famous and having a million-dollar mansion. I'm talking about living the life that you can afford right now, in the space that you're in.

Did you know that if you take this dream and break it down into actionable steps, you have an achievable goal? When you take one step at a time consistently, your goal will become a reality before you know it. You can use this plan with almost anything: weight loss, writing a book, running a marathon, tidying your house, working on your relationships and all those sorts of things. Goal setting can be quite easy, especially when the overthinking is removed.

What I know for sure is that if you don't pay attention to your Kefi Future, you will live a life of regret. When you're on your death bed and you look back over your life, are you going to see broken dreams, regrets and no legacy or connection?

It has been said that at the end of life, many people regret the things that they didn't do. Losing weight to be healthier is a big one. Staying in their dead-end unfulfilling job is another. Also not spending time with the family, foregoing holidays and experiences and staying at work from morning till dark. How do you want it to be for you?

So, look at those memories and legacies. What is it that you wish to achieve?

After I separated, for the next few years I still didn't have the clarity I was looking for. My kefi was missing; I'd totally forgotten that I had once known what it was to be happy and fulfilled, to have hopes and dreams and to understand how to achieve them. The next ten years were pivotal, as it was easy to see how things didn't get easier after I separated because of the way that I was. It wasn't until I engaged in a lot of personal development processes that I was able rebuild myself to where I am today.

One day I was talking to a new friend, who was running a program and had a clear vision of what he wanted to do and who he wanted to help. He turned to me and said after explaining his dreams for three hours, 'So what are your dreams?'

I stopped dead in my tracks. 'I'm not really sure, oh, ah, err …' I then understood that I didn't have any dreams. I was walking through life in a daze after the trauma of everyday life. Nothing monumental in particular, but small things: disappointment, broken dreams, failure, sadness, heartache, grief, that sort of stuff.

From that moment in 2007 I realised I needed to review what I was doing and start learning more about what I wanted, although I wasn't quite sure how to do it at that point. I've always been an over-thinker so I often didn't take the steps that I needed to take. Many times, I started diets. I could write a PhD on the weight loss books I have read. I probably could buy a whole house on the amount of investment I have put into programs, gyms, health food, appointments — trying to find the magic pill to make it right.

However, when no one was watching, no matter what I was doing and saying in public, I was still sneaking lollies, cakes, biscuits and a bit of baklava here and there. I didn't take any simple consistent steps towards my goals, my future — I was going round in circles.

I was not looking into the future. I've had a couple of health issues, mainly due to my lack of taking action steps. Things are changing for me on that front, as I take action every day: simple things like walking for an hour most days (and a big one in not eating ice cream, which fed my inner child).

I can see how I want my future to be. I know I want to travel to Greece more often. I know I wish to be slimmer and fitter; I'm working on that.

I know that I want to attract a new partner into my life. But I won't settle this time around, so I'm being very cautious and picky with what I won't put up with and who I choose to hang out with.

What I do know for sure is that any time I've achieved huge success, I got some professional assistance. I've employed coaches along the way and mentors who've helped me with quite a lot of what I've needed to do. I gained the clarity, the know-how and the drive to take action, without thinking too much about it.

This coaching really helped me with how to get clear on what I really wanted. Even though I knew that I wanted something different, I still wasn't 100% sure of what I wanted. I've heard of the vision board process, envisaging what you want to look like and who you want to attract and all these things, but I didn't really believe it and didn't really feel it in my heart.

The coaches I've worked with have all helped me in some way, shape or form. I had lots of friends who were coaches, but they couldn't quite get me past where I was – so I was still infinitely stuck in a process of trying to change, but not quite getting there, never truly believing that I could change.

Believing is achieving; believing is where it starts. One particular coach said to me as we were talking, 'You always tell stories about other people. You never really say what you think.' It wasn't until that 'ah ha' moment that I saw that I needed to really start dropping into my body and understanding what I wanted for me.

Kefi Future is all about what you want for you, first and foremost — and then how it impacts on the people around you.

So many people who I work with talk about not knowing what they want ... I didn't know what I wanted for so long. Now I have absolute clarity. After trauma in your life, you can feel like you're a zombie and you're just going through the motions. Getting in touch with your values and beliefs makes a difference, so start with the small steps. Understand who you are and what you want. Understand that you can have more than what you're accepting right now. But you've got to plan for it; saying 'I want a new job' and then waiting for the new job to fall in your lap is just not going to cut it. You just have to do something to make it happen. If you don't read the paper to see if there are any jobs, or you don't go online to where the job agency is advertising their positions, if you don't ask around — if you don't even have a current CV — all those things won't work.

So many people also tell me that 'goals never work for me'. Sometimes the goals that you set are actually set too far into the future. Sometimes I just ask, 'Well what do you want?'

So you want to be able to clean and declutter your world? Start with your wallet or handbag. Put the timer on for fifteen minutes. Get some help, get into the garden and clear the mess. What are you waiting for?

Take some small action steps where you can move more every day. Maybe it's going swimming or going to a dance class. If you don't actually do the things you know that you want (or need) to do, you will never achieve your goals. It's not going to come to you by magic (Appendix 2).

So often people tell me they hate their job, their house, their shape – partner or mother or father ... 'I hate my life, I hate, hate, hate, hate!'

If nothing changes, nothing changes. Just think about that for a moment. If you keep doing the things that you're doing, you're going to stay in the same position and your kefi is just going to remain hidden inside of you. It's going to stay locked away instead of coming out and allowing you to celebrate the things that you want.

Three action steps you can take as a result of reading Kefi Future:

1) Take time to imagine yourself in one year's time. Project into your future and think about where you wish to be. Write about how your life is at that point: how you'll feel, what you'll be thinking, what you'll see and hear. What do you wish to achieve? The big focus is on how you will feel at this time.

2) Create a vision board. Collect images from magazines or go online to build a picture of how you want your house to look, how you will live your life or how you want to feel. Those are the things that you can keep as a visual reminder every day.

3) You can use a SMART goals template to write a kefi bucket list. Often people don't know what they want and don't know where to go with it all. So, they find it a challenge. You will find it useful to focus on each Column of Strength for inspiration for your future goals.

What I would suggest is to focus hard on what it is that you want, because you can have that kefi life. The Kefi Future of your dreams.

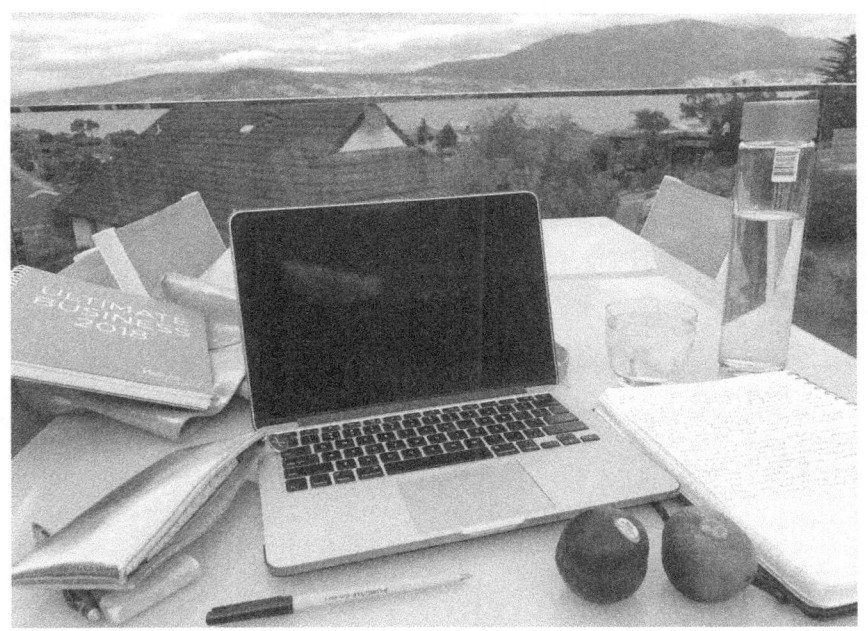

Chapter 7

Kefi Fortune

'Wealth consists not in having great possessions, but in having few wants.'
– **Epictetus, philosopher**

'Not what we have, but what we enjoy constitutes our abundance.'
– **Epicurus, philosopher**

The Bible says, 'For the love of money is the root of all kinds of evils' (Timothy 6:10). It just causes so many problems, as having enough isn't always enough for some people. 'How you do money is how you do life' is another common saying. What you do with your spending can have a huge impact on how you live your life in the future.

Having a Kefi Fortune means that you have enough money to do what you want when you want – without the struggle and without the stress of not having enough. It's not just referring to money: it's also about gratitude and seeing that you have a good life, one that celebrates feeling fortunate.

Often, I have heard as I was growing up how I had champagne tastes on a beer income, or that I'd need to marry a millionaire to keep the life I was accustomed to. Perhaps it was to keep me grounded and realistic about money.

Every person has the opportunity to live the way that they wish to live, according to their income. An income basically comes from the type of work that you do. When your work, your passion and your kefi all match up, then you'll find that you have enough money for whatever it is that you need. Sometimes the need to spend ('retail therapy') is actually about emotions or core needs that are not being met. Overspending creates other issues and impacts so many other things – which I experienced first hand a few years ago.

Being aware of your buying strategy and how you spend is pure gold. If you know that you're going into a store and you just can't resist the sales, so you end up putting more on your credit card, is that the best strategy for your bank balance – especially for something that you perhaps may not need? Or do you invest in high end programs, thinking it will give you what you need to get your business up off the ground? Does your decision end up stretching your budget so that it is a catalyst for arguments with your husband or partner?

So often you see people purchasing their winter wardrobe or their summer wardrobe all in one hit, and then they don't go shopping again until the following season. That can be of benefit, because you don't have the impulse buying issue. It always amazed me when I heard stories like this, as many women I know list shopping as a hobby.

Quite often the issue of impulse buying can have an impact on the way that you manage money. Where do you invest your income? How do you invest in yourself? How do you grow as a person?

Kefi Fortune isn't just about money, however – it's also about how you feel wealthy, empowered and energised in your life. When you feel fortunate, you feel the most fulfilling gratitude. When you experience Kefi Fortune, you are grateful for everything and you live your life with grace.

The benefit of Kefi Fortune is that you live life with a wealth mindset. Mindset is so important; everything revolves around it. Being able to feel rich in all areas of your life is also a very important thing. When you understand how you interact with money then it becomes easier to reflect on your spending, to understand what it is that you do.

I know lots of people do online shopping now. Many people

have said to me that they've actually saved money by not going into a supermarket, because they don't impulse buy sales or things that they see at the end of the aisle; they find that they only buy the things that they absolutely need. Therefore, they're not spending on the extras jumping into the shopping trolley.

Consciously being aware of your money mindset, and of how you feel fortunate and grateful in your life, can be built up in a conscious manner. Focus on what you do have rather than what you do not. Rather than saying you can't afford to buy something, look at it another way: 'How can I afford to buy the thing I desire?'

By raising your awareness, you can actually do something about it. If you feel that you can't afford things, then it's time to review your spending. Look inside your wallet or purse so you know how much you've got. Or do you only use a plastic card to pay for everything?

The shocking truth is that money is tricky. Everyone needs it and there's more than enough to go around. So often we are told that we need more – we have to work harder and accumulate more stuff. We have become a disposable society in a very short time. Not everything is used up. When we get tired of something, we replace it (even if it is not worn out). How often are we shown the line-up of people desperate for the latest technology such as phones and gaming platforms? The previous one still works but the marketing strategies are so powerful people can't resist. We hear that we can spend now and pay later. What happened to saving up?

The click and go modern age is dictating the methods used to spend money. There is a 'need it right away' mentality that is evident in so many areas of society. At the risk of showing my age – in my day when I was young, we had to save and put money in our bankbook before we could even consider buying a biggish ticket item.

But money can be really elusive at times and it feels as if you never have enough. Marketing has us wanting more: more stuff, more experiences, more, more, more. At what cost? How does it impact on the stress and strain of making ends meet?

I often hear that there isn't enough money coming in. When we look more closely, however, there *is* enough coming in – the focus on outgoing expenses evaluates how it all doesn't balance. There is no talk of balancing the chequebook or the cash register at the end of the day.

Do you feel that you're on the treadmill of catch-up, going from paycheque to paycheque, never having enough to pay the last month's bills and not quite enough to be able to save for the future? Do you find that it causes arguments between you and your partner? Are you stressed? Do you feel that you're broke all the time? Are you living in a scarcity mindset, where there's never enough and you just feel like there's poverty around you? They're the things that you can look at to work out strategies to create a change.

Money causes so many issues for people, as everyone's relationship with money is very different. There is talk of wealth and how much things cost, buying stuff you don't need. It can even be a feeling of euphoria when you make that purchase: the new dress, top, shoes, jewellery, makeup, accessory and so on.

When you don't feel like you're wealthy or that things are going well – when you feel that it's all beyond you – it's really challenging to feel that you're fortunate and that there's any kefi going on around you. I've quite a bit of experience in this area.

I was burnt out and quit teaching a few years back. I felt undervalued and overworked and I just wasn't in a good place. It wasn't long until life had changed and I moved into the city, away from the life that I had before. I had my children with me every second week and they were with their father every other week. I was learning to adjust to quite a number of things.

My Kefi Fortune seemed totally out of whack; I felt I never had enough money. My body would clench up and I felt my stomach churn every time I opened a bill. I was consumed by feelings of lack and fear. I couldn't see how I was going to improve my lot and have a life. I stopped spending on entertainment for myself. I never went to the movies, out to dinner with friends – even coffee was a stretch. I hardly ever bought clothes for myself. I felt frumpy and used food to medicate my feelings all over again.

By making changes in the way that I operated, changing the places that I went to and where I worked, I could make new choices for myself and change my story. There was a lot of risk involved and I had to shake my tree, to let go of control and wanting to know what was happening next. I had trust and faith that I would get work, be able to pay my bills and put food on the table for my kids.

What I found was even though I was passionate about teaching and I loved what was going on in the workplace and the classroom, the institutional nature of the school just didn't suit me anymore. Twenty-four years of this daily grind had me stressed and burnt out. I also found that I hated meetings, marking and the after-hours work with a passion, because I just couldn't balance it all with the rest of my life. My Kefi Fortune needed a shake-up as I wasn't feeling very fortunate at all.

My credit card also got out of control. Because I was now a relief teacher, I didn't have employment during the school holidays. To make matters worse, I was not in the space where I actually saved ahead of time for the holidays. In the end, I had no money left for the holidays, because I also had to pay my mortgage with credit. I actually had more than one credit card; there were two or three, plus a store card. The total value of my credit card debt was $23,000. For some people that may not sound like a lot of money, but I was a single parent working intermittently as a relief teacher and I had no idea how I could get myself out of the mess that I'd gotten myself into. I am not quite sure how I gathered so many cards in my purse!

Along the way, I understood that I needed to do something about it and fear got the better of me. My body tensed up; I had a sore neck, my lower back ached and my heels became swollen so it was hard to walk. Your body is a barometer and shows you when something is not right!

My fear was off the charts. The unknown and potential loss was circling like a shark. I had no idea what I should do to sort the financial mess I was in. When I couldn't meet my mortgage repayment, I knew I had to do something different. I couldn't bury my head in the sand any more. I went and saw my trusted friend, showing him all of my documents and confessing to all of my debts. I was in a real pickle. He listened intensely to all I had to say, and then stopped to think for a moment. I could see that he was struggling with what he was about to say. He advised me to sell my house and move in with my mum after I had paid off all my debts. Simple, really.

What I did after that was extremely empowering. It felt like it was the end of the world at the time. However, from that I came to understand more about the way I handle money. First, I reviewed my finances and created a budget. The budget is the most important thing I have done and I've gone through this process more than once now. It's really important to understand how much I need to pay my bills and meet my outgoings, as well as being able to put food on the table, petrol in my car and have a little bit of entertainment.

That budget was the turning point for my finances. After I cut up my credit cards, I started to use only cash or a debit card to pay for purchases. That was huge. Embroiled in all of that was my lack of ability to make decisions for myself and to trust the decisions I was making. I learnt that by listening to myself and trusting myself to make decisions for me and my kids, I broke free of the past in when I was burnt by past experiences.

All in all, I turned my life around in twenty-one days – from the time I went to see my trusted friend and getting my house ready to go to market. It came about because my mother, sister and cousin rallied around to help me (my Kefi Family). I then signed off with an agent to put my house on the market – the sign was up for a few days and before I knew it, I had a signed contract and a very short settlement. It took twenty-one days to make the decision and to have the signed contract in my hand. It was a whirlwind.

As I moved into my Kefi Chicks business, defining who I was and what I believed in, I found it really challenging to feel my value, because I wanted to give everything I learnt away for free. However, this was not going to help the fortunes of my family; I understood that I was investing in myself and that by sharing my knowledge, I was able to empower other people and share with them the things that I'd learnt. Kefi Chicks was born around the same time I made the decision to sell my house.

By paying attention to where you're spending your money, you start seeing that you might be spending it on things that are really unnecessary. Do you need to go out for breakfast? Do you take lunch to work? What things do you do that are necessary and which things are unnecessary?

It's quite easy to create a budget, use this one in Appendix 1 of this book to get started. A budget will allow you and your family to understand what you spend your money on, and more importantly how much you need to earn. So often people tell me they never have any money. Well, this is your chance to become your own money detective to unpack what you are doing with it.

Quite simply, list all of the things you need to pay each fortnight or month: electricity, phone, water, insurance, mortgage, car repayments, any other outgoings that you know and expect. Then focus on how much you spend on food at the supermarket, eating out, incidentals, clothes, haircuts, gifts, maintenance – list it all and work out how much you need to bring in. Old bank statements can be helpful with this process.

Until you watch your spending habits and really focus your attention, how will you know where your money goes? How will you know how you spend it? How will you know what it is that you do?

Many times when I've been talking to people who wish to invest in themselves, they tell me, 'I can't afford to do that,' or, 'I have to ask my husband.' What is the cost of this to you? What is this money mindset that you're pursuing? What are you teaching your kids about never having enough? If you only make decisions with your husband's say-so, sometimes it takes away your power and freedom. It doesn't allow you to be kind to yourself — to empower yourself and be inspired to be more. Look for ways you can invest in yourself to be a better version of yourself, for you and future generations.

Of course, you're going to need to talk to your partner about your budget and spending as a family. That is the right thing to do. However, empowering yourself to make decisions and to be able to invest in yourself is something that is going to give you so much more than you ever imagined.

In the previous chapter, we talked about Kefi Future. This chapter goes right along with it. Understanding your Kefi Fortune, and how your finances impacts on your whole way of being, will make a huge difference in the way that you see yourself and your world.

Three action steps you can take as a result of reading Kefi Fortune:

1) Understand your spending habits by doing your budget. Knowing where your money goes can be empowering. Work out how much you need to pay your expenses and then see what is left over. Understand what you do, find out what you want to change and stick to the plan.

2) Journal about how you manage money; observe your spending habits and buying strategy. Do you have any beliefs which impact on how you spend or save money? What is your first memory around money? There is so much emotion when people talk about money. How does money make you feel?

3) Clear your clutter and develop a system. Clean out your wallet and handbag. Put all your bills in one place. Keep an eye on your bank statements. Know what you can spend. Have a savings plan so you can afford to indulge or go on holiday. Being organised in this way will make a difference.

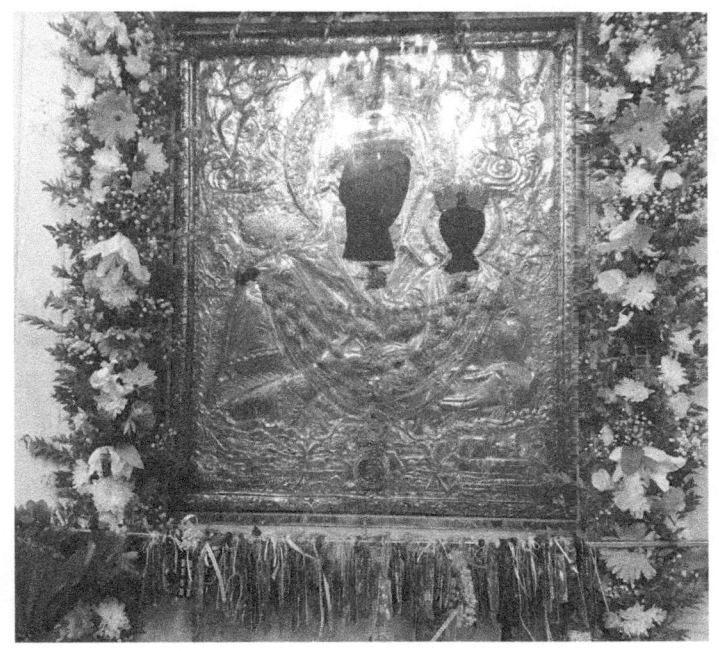

Chapter 8

Kefi Faith

'Truly I tell you, if you have faith as small as a mustard seed, you can say to this mountain, "Move from here to there," and it will move. Nothing will be impossible for you.'
– Matthew 17:20, New International Version (NIV)

'Our prayers should be for blessings in general, for God knows best what is good for us.'
– Socrates, philosopher

A spiritual practice steeped in the traditions of the Greek Orthodox faith can provide peace, self-love and balance. Embracing Kefi Faith is having a spiritual practice based on the teaching and learnings of the Greek Orthodox faith. It is a very strong Column of Strength which provides a moral compass and the elements known to enhance a person's life and way of being. It is steeped in our tradition, culture and heritage with how we interact and how we do things.

There are many benefits of having a spiritual practice. Not everyone is connected to the same faith. When I'm talking about spiritual practice, I'm going to be referring to my experience in the Greek Orthodox faith and how I went on a journey of self-discovery to come full circle, returning to something that I've found gave me peace, connection, grace and harmony. It helped me be the person I am today. It helped me clear my head and it also helped me understand myself further.

Some benefits of a spiritual practice of having a strong, Kefi Faith is that it promotes hope and optimism. The studies as mentioned by Clay Routledge PhD have proven that people who are connected to a faith or a religion do find that it promotes hope and feelings of wellbeing[2]. Currently there are lots of different schools of thought on this and it is going to be important for you to determine how this works for your family. This connection to a Greek way of life must not be underestimated.

---

2   Routledge, C 2014, '5 Scientifically Supported Benefits of Prayer', *Psychology Today*, <https://www.psychologytoday.com/blog/more-mortal/201406/5-scientifically-supported-benefits-prayer>.

Having connection and a sense of self-belonging is really powerful for the whole family, because it brings people together in a way that has happened in many cultures in many different ways. In the Greek Orthodox faith, being able to belong is very important for many people. Ideally, it also builds a belief in yourself. It boosts self-esteem, because believing in a higher power allows you to be that person who can see there is good in the world. It is soothing to the spirit and to your soul when you are involved in a spiritual practice.

Kefi Faith is very strong on helping people develop inner peace and presence. When you are present in your world, every day, you notice what's going on; you see and feel and know that this is important for you.

Love is not a feeling – love is faith in action. Quite a lot of people are finding that they are disconnected from feelings of love. When you have faith, you know that love is central to everything and from that flows happiness.

The Kefi Faith Column of Strength is pivotal and essential to be able to get your kefi back.

Without kefi in the area of faith, people are sceptical. There is a lack of connection, there's no tribe and there's a lack of self-worth. A church is a place of communion, a place where there is connection. It assists you to connect with yourself and removes the distractions that are placed in your way on a daily basis.

Faith is the belief in an innate power greater than yourself. It becomes part of you and integrates into every Column of Strength. It completes you and is part of a whole. It enhances connection on a daily basis with yourself and others. Too often I hear the confusion of people criticising the patriarchal system of the church or the politics which are part and parcel of any organisation. This has, in reality, no part to play in how you develop your Kefi Faith.

Connected, these are the initial elements of the Greek Orthodox faith. Many people focus on the things that they dislike when they go to a church. What I've come to understand after a soul-searching journey of self-discovery, through some other spiritual practices that were certainly in no way part of who I am today, is that the answer can be so simple. I was trying to make my life better, at a time when I was looking to find a solution to my problems in my married life; I went along to a group which in the end was most certainly not for my highest good.

I was so disconnected from my family, myself and my traditions, culture and heritage that I was lost and totally alone. I became drawn to a spiritual teacher who taught me things that went against my identity, culture, and traditions – these things don't match. Instead of things getting better, they got worse. After I separated, I moved towards my faith once again and the healing process began in earnest.

I've found that returning to my Greek faith was the thing that really assisted my self-healing. The church was a place where I came to pray, focus myself and be me. A place to let go of the hurt and the pain. A place of healing.

My journey back to church taught me to find inner peace and connection. I was no longer lost, and I was much more hopeful of finding happiness. I cleared my home of all things which were not part of my Greek Orthodox faith and focused on embracing what I have known from a child, when I would go to church mostly with my *yiayia* (grandmother). My parents were working seven days a week in their grocery store and rarely got to take a break.

I started to feel whole, I started to know that I was in my place, in my place of comfort, my soul was being nourished and I was feeling so much better. I found that going to church every Sunday was something I just had to do. My friends would say to me that their mothers had seen me again in church. Their mothers wanted to encourage their daughters to follow my lead and kept repeating that they saw me. One even said, 'Can you stop going? My mother is harassing me!' My reply was that I was doing this for me and not anyone else – what they did was their choice.

I learnt that I needed to go back to my roots. I found that by connecting with people at church – by helping out with things like the Easter *epitafio* (Christ's tomb), seeing people regularly, going for coffee with my new friends on a regular basis with people that I met at church – I empowered my feelings of connection and love. My friends would share their understandings and I asked questions. I received gifts of prayer books and the liturgy from members of the congregation, who were thrilled to welcome me to the fold. I was gifted the rather large volume of Easter services, which was in both English and Greek, and helped me follow along and understand what was going on. Growing up Greek, I had never understood what was going on in church.

It is common practice for children to be baptised or christened when they are babies. A baptism is a central sacrament in a Greek family. A Good Greek Girl marries in the Greek Orthodox church, and christens her children in the right way at the right time. I had not done any of these things and it did not sit well with me. I had always dreamed that I would get married in our local Greek church to a Greek man and we would live happily ever after. None of this was to be.

I had my children baptised after a trip to Greece in 2010, because they weren't baptised from a young age. I had said to my mum that it would be great if we could get them christened when we were in Greece. I had no sooner returned when I bumped into a friend (at Officeworks of all places) and we proceeded to have this amazing conversation about it. Without a second thought she said, 'I will be a *nona* to your daughter.'

I visited her with my son and daughter and my friend quickly hit it off with my thirteen year old son. She became his *nona* and her husband became my daughter's *nono*. It was a big family affair and I felt something calm within after this. I felt I had found a way to protect my children as it didn't feel right on a spiritual level not to have them embraced by my Kefi Faith.

It provides family connections when people are your best man or woman, when you become a *koumbara* or *koumbaros* (an Orthodox sponsor). When you are the *nona* or *nono* (godparent) to someone's children they become part of your Kefi Family. Both of those are a big deal in Kefi Faith, with important benefits and obligations to maintain a connection for spiritual practices within the family. As a baby there is a baptism or christening, which is a Sacrament; the child's rebirth is celebrated together with the new relationship with their godparent, who is responsible for the child on a spiritual level.

I was eleven when I became a *nona* for a gorgeous girl, whom I have always been there for. I have taken my duties as a godparent very seriously and have discussed the things I know are part of the Greek Orthodox way of life: regular church attendance, confession, communion, lighting your *kandili* (it represents the light of Christ in the home), prayer and so much more, including connecting with your local priest.

The *kandili* or vigil lamp is a reminder to slow down; it acts as a place to shut out the world and enter into a state of peace. I keep mine in a corner of my kitchen and have some icons near it. My *kandili* is made out of glass. I place a small amount of water in the bottom and then add light olive oil on top. I use '*fitilakia*', which is a wick floating attached to a thin piece of cork – I get this from church. This then floats on top of the oil. When I get up in the morning it is one of the places I pray before I start my day.

When I reconnected with my Kefi Faith by attending church regularly, I made new friends and my family expanded. Because I was in the right place, it felt natural – and it feels to this very day like a place that's for me. Each person needs to go through their own journey and to find out what's right for them. It is where I find community and a sense of belonging.

I didn't grow up with a *kandili* in our house or with the house being incensed on a regular basis, but that's now part of my daily and weekly practice so that I'm able to keep my house clear and light – that way it feels like I'm energised when I'm in my home space.

I found that I was embracing a spiritual practice that aligned with my culture, traditions and heritage and it felt right.

The healing of my heart was certainly something that kept developing each time. I don't know if you've ever seen the icon of the Panagia (Virgin Mary) with the seven swords. She has seven swords, three from each side and one from down below all pointing into her heart, which are symbolic of her pain and suffering with her son Jesus being crucified. It certainly resonates with me and how I once felt about things.

Kefi Faith is an empowering and freeing Column of Strength. Learning to go with the flow is really powerful. Let go of control. Stop trying to get everyone organised; stop being the teacher, the director of traffic and behaviour. Learn to live in the now. Quieten your mind and stop forcing things. I know my broken heart allowed me to be vulnerable and to trust again. The pain and suffering that I thought I was going through, the story that I was stuck in, was only from my perspective. I told myself lots and lots of stories of what was done to me along the way and slowly but surely, I allowed those things to be released. I changed my story. You can too. Awareness is key; watch what you do so you can implement small behavioural changes.

Kefi Faith is very, very powerful and it cannot be underestimated. The spiritual practices of your childhood may be very different to the ones that I'm referring to today. Quite often people say that they don't go to church. One of my friend's mothers used to say, 'If you drive past a friend's place, you go in and visit them, don't you? If you're driving past a church and you don't go in and visit your friend God, what sort of friend are you?' That always stuck with me. Another of my friend's mum always said, 'You give up time to go out to do other things, why can't you give up some time to go to church?'

Another thing I get told: 'My partner and family don't follow Greek Orthodox ways.' Following the practice that works for you is the crucial part here. You do what is right for you: go to church, fast when you can, have communion, pray, read, immerse yourself in Kefi Faith. Do what is right for you.

The Sacrament of Holy Communion is an integral part of Kefi Faith and the Greek Orthodox faith. This is a way to remember Jesus Christ. Preparation is required prior to receiving Holy Communion, including fasting and confession. I used to think confession was really scary and my first two experiences certainly lived up to that. My first time was with a monk from Mt Athos who spoke no English; I was so stressed my Greek didn't come out very well. The first thing I spoke of was that I didn't get married in the Greek Orthodox Church, which was very heavy – his reaction was total shock. It just about had me running out the church door never to return.

In due course, my chats with my local priests have been empowering and have me delving deeper into how and why I do certain things. Each time after a discussion or confession, I kneel under the *epitrachelion (stole)* of the priest who then says a prayer.

During my most recent visit only a couple of weeks ago, the priest shared a story with me. He spoke of a village of people who lived around the edge of a frozen lake. The people need to get to the other side to go about their daily lives. The people think nothing of crossing a frozen lake, which can be perceived to be dangerous. The greatest tendency is to get to the other side as quickly as possible without ever cutting a hole in the ice to have a look beneath the surface. Under the surface there is a whole other world. It is when you look beneath the surface that you find the things that matter so you can put them in perspective.

In Kefi Faith it is part of the process to cut a hole in the ice to discover the things that matter. Prayer, regular church attendance, understand and learning about Orthodoxy. It assists with the healing process and is not a scary or difficult process; in fact, it is liberating and empowering.

After visiting the priest it is one of the best times to partake in Holy Communion.

Quite often people tell me they don't fast at Easter time or Christmas time, or during the year. They fast for a few days beforehand only. I changed my daily practices as I came to understand more about my faith, so that I refrain from meat and animal products on a Wednesday and a Friday, rather than having a big lead up. I also attend church most Sundays, occasionally I find that I don't get there. But it's a rare occasion.

After church, I hang out with my church friends and the ladies who make coffee and cakes and things like that. We work as a community and when you are with the people who you see as your tribe, things feel right. I know this because when I was married, I didn't marry somebody with my set of values and cultural influences, and things were very different and challenging.

When I went to Greece recently, I was fortunate enough to go to Meteora. There are places in the world that create a sense of inner peace – a stillness that allows you to hear yourself, to feel free and to release those negative thoughts that keep you stuck in the same old story. Meteora is one of those places – it's a spiritual place. It is one of the largest and most important complexes of monasteries in all of Greece, second only to Mt Athos. It's possible to do a tour or you can take yourself there and visit different monasteries.

I love collecting icons and I have a collection on display in a cabinet that was once my mother's in my home. I have some in almost every room of my home. I have collected them from a variety of places – some I bought in Greece on two different trips, some from the churches I have visited, and some have been given to me as gifts. One of my favourites is the icon my grandmother brought with her for Greece almost 100 years ago of the Panagia Myrtidiotissa from the island of Kythera.

One of the reasons for my most recent visit to Greece was to be in Kythera on 24 September for the honouring of this icon. The year before my mother passed we were decorating this icon for the service in Hobart and I said to her that I would like to be in Kythera next year for this celebration. I was not to know that I was going to be there a year later.

Finding spiritual peace from chaos is a wonderful thing. There are lots of monasteries and churches in Greece (and in many other places around the world) where you can discover the truth for yourself, find that peace and learn about service for the people. So many people tell me that they haven't got time to go to church. What I know to be true for me is that this is where the real healing happens: the letting go, the rebuilding and strengthening of you as a person.

Kefi Faith is focused on reclaiming your traditions, culture and heritage to connect (or reconnect) on a deeper level so that you can pay it all forward and enhance someone else's life.

I also hear from people, 'I don't know how to start.' Spiritual practice starts with you and the first step is attending church. Connect with your local priest; some churches have Bible study classes and lectures, which is a great place to start. Visit your *yiayia*, mother, aunt or family friend who already is involved and talk about the things that are important in the life of the church.

Light candles. You may like to light a *kandili* to incense your home; you may find yourself reading the Bible or other appropriate books more, talking to people who understand the spiritual ways of Greek Orthodoxy. When the student is ready, the teacher will appear.

By reconnecting or deepening your connection to Kefi Faith you will:

- learn to deal with stress more effectively
- release reserves of untapped energies
- transform anger
- heal relationships
- leave behind painful memories
- live a life fully in the present
- develop insight and understanding
- learn to love more fully than though possible
- discover your contribution to life.

There are many places you can look and many people who can assist you. Be open to the process and God will provide.

Three action steps you can take as a result of reading Kefi Faith:

1) Visit your local church and light a candle. When was the last time you visited a church? Give thanks as you light your candle. Attend a church liturgy and participate in the sacraments. Make an appointment to speak to your local priest to get things off your chest and to have a blessing.

2) Reflect on how you learnt about faith as a young child. Did you go to church as a child? When, which church and with whom? What's different now? What's the same? Do you wear your christening cross? Do you have any icons? You may like to purchase one of the saint you were named after.

3) Create a sacred space in your home to place an icon or two and a *kandili*. Consider where you can offer to be kind to others in your home, family and friends to start with. What is the tone you wish to set in your home spiritually? What example are you setting for others?

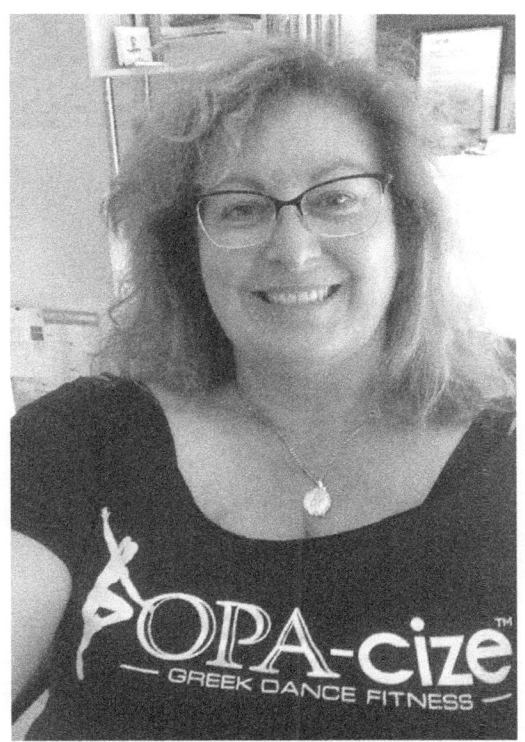

Chapter 9

Kefi Fit

'Let him that would move the world first move himself.'
— **Socrates, philosopher**

'Life must be lived as play.'
— **Plato, philosopher**

Greeks love to party and are up on the dance floor as soon as they hear their favourite song. Dancing is inclusive and no partner is required. There's nothing like a fun-filled fitness program to get your heart pumping. We all know what we should be doing; it is taking action that becomes the challenge.

Kefi Fit is all about moving your body, doing the things that you know will increase your health benefits and getting you the results that you're looking for. It encompasses more than just a fit body — a fit mind and spirit (or soul) also sit here.

There's nothing better than feeling great about yourself, knowing that your body is steeled with strength and power. As we get older, we know that the health benefits of being fit is paramount. I'm preaching to the converted here, I'm sure. So how is it that we hear that obesity is on the rise, along with all the related health issues?

Another benefit of being Kefi Fit is that you have a calm state of mind, so those things that get to you when you're feeling fragile or under the pump don't affect you as much as they would normally when you're not so fit.

Being Kefi Fit means that you're focused and you get things done; you get on with the job and stop procrastinating. It means to avoid being overwhelmed and reduce your stress. It means you get active and move your body as a non-negotiable activity on a daily basis.

How awesome is that? It's a well known fact that getting active helps you achieve your goals. Sixty per cent of gym memberships go unused according to Statistic Brain[3]. Rather than running out and getting a gym membership, look around and find out what's available to you. How many times have you invested in a gym membership, only to go a few times and then life gets in the way?

If you're in the unhealthy weight range and not moving much at all, you risk diabetes, heart attacks and high blood pressure to name but a few. Being Kefi Fit is so much more empowering. When stuff happens, it is so easy to stop doing the things that matter, to become sedentary and to overeat. Especially when life gets you down and your mindset works against you. Being Kefi Fit means moving your body in ways which include fun and laughter. It is effortless and you don't have to talk yourself into moving.

Raise your hand if you are guilty of being a member of a gym, which you didn't visit. Raise your hand if you overthink all of the things that you should be doing, such as walking, swimming, jogging or lifting some weights, but the actions never happen. Raise your hand if you are looking for the magic pill to make it happen without doing any of the work. I know just how that feels too.

Have you convinced yourself it's your genes that keep you looking the way that you do? Are you in denial about your size? Do you pretend to accept how unfit you are, or the way you look? Do you laugh it off when you get told you look pregnant when you're not? These are things I know to be true for me as well as a number of clients I have worked with. Over ten years ago I remember saying to someone that I didn't want to look how I did back then at forty; I wanted to be trim, taught and terrific. I wanted it on a mental level but I wasn't prepared

---

3   Statistic Brain 2017, 'Gym Membership Statistics', <https://www.statisticbrain.com/gym-membership-statistics/>.

to do the work and change my eating enough to make the difference I was looking for.

It can be such a vicious circle. You beat yourself up because you put on weight again and you can't fit into your clothes, so you spiral down into negative self-talk. You feel fat and frumpy and you avoid being seen in anything except layers of black clothing, as that at least makes you look slimmer. The bedroom is a place where you avoid any physical contact because you believe your self-talk about not being attractive to anyone, let alone yourself. It can play havoc on your marriage and relationships.

Being Kefi Fit is so much more than just your body; it's also about the mind. When you're physically fit, your mindset is also fit. It comes along for the ride, because when you exercise you release endorphins and other magical hormones and chemicals, which all contribute to feeling good.

Knowing the outcome you desire is only one part of the story. Quite often it is common to know what you want and to have a general idea of how to get it. It can all come unstuck in a very short time because you want quick results. The gentle reminder is that it took quite a number of years to look the way you do now, so it is not going to be a quick fix that will get you the results. Also, we have been schooled to believe that massive effort is required: food and exercise programs exist in abundance. So why are so many not working on a long term basis?

In my experience, small changes can bring big results on a long term basis. I've spent large amounts of money in the past looking for a quick fix, which required so much mental energy and focus that my mindset was to pack it in early. Having the ability to notice what's working and what isn't – as well as being flexible to make changes as you need to remain informed by the results that you are getting – is where the gold begins.

Small steps, even baby steps will get you there. After going around in circles and looping for so many years, my non-negotiables are walking for an hour every day and not eating ice cream. I also trained as a Greek Dance Fitness instructor, as I knew that my kefi would go through the roof inspiring other women while dancing.

And how great is it to always feel good and to build your kefi so that it influences all areas of your life? The comparison trap that we can fall into is about body shaming and feeling guilty about the way we look – all of those things that Good Greek Girls talk themselves into, coming down from generational thinking. This needs to be shattered. We have to feel good from within first, so that the world can see those changes on the outside.

I don't want my daughter or her friends, or my nieces or granddaughters (should I be fortunate enough to have any), to feel the way that I have at times. I never want them to feel ashamed of their body. I never want them to know what it's like to be called fat. I never want them to feel embarrassed of their body or the way they look. I want them to be the person they're supposed to be because of who they are, not what they look like.

The way a person looks does not define who they are. The comparison trap takes us to the place where we do not match up to the way the media represents models in magazines or films. It is not possible to match up to the ideal look of a size 2 model or a size 0 model who doesn't eat and does not live life the way a Kefi Chick should. I don't want that for any woman anywhere, anytime! It is not okay.

Too often people fail at losing weight. Too often the weight loss industry is happy to take the money, but the results don't match the expenditure. What I know for sure is small steps start with regular, manageable exercise. Forget about the food for the first part. That comes in a following chapter. We're looking to find how you can become fitter, healthier and more active in your twilight years.

I've had frequent gym memberships. In the most part, my money has been a donation to the gym and I'd go a few times and then I wouldn't be seen again. A few years would pass, I'd go and join another gym and so on, until I worked out that it was time to stop spending money on something that I just wasn't using.

A few years ago, a new dance craze came to Hobart: Zumba. It was amazing. I love to dance: it's high-energy, fun and it got me fit. Did it change my whole body size? No. But I did feel that I was able to achieve anything that I wanted to. It got me out of my head and into my body, and that's why dancing is so amazing. After a few years I stopped taking Zumba classes and teaching it in schools when I was doing relief. Slowly but surely, more weight piled on and I stopped feeling great about myself again.

My most recent foray into exercise is to become a Greek Dance Fitness class instructor. Greek Dance Fitness classes are taking off right now; they're everything a Kefi Chick needs. It has Greek music pumping, uses classic Greek dance moves, you are surrounded by other Greek women (or women who also love to dance) – it is a great recipe for success. It's going to get you Kefi Fit.

If you aren't able to get to a Greek Dance Fitness class, I suggest that you put some music on and dance around anywhere that you choose, with or without other people, and crank it up really loud – just enjoy it. There is no hard and fast rule on how you should do this and there is no right or wrong way to dance. There is no judgement; just get out there and do it. That's what I've found has made a huge difference and I'm finding that things have changed in my body because of it.

For a while, I also became a regular swimmer. I was never a good swimmer. Swimming was not my first love when it came to any sort of exercise, unless it was a hot day or at the beach.

I was working with a mentor just out of Port Macquarie a few years ago and there was a pool at the apartment block where I was staying. It was warm and sunny, so I got in the pool, despite my size – I ignored and shoved down those feelings, and the impact on my health was enormous. I had found something I loved, and my body didn't ache and groan afterwards. When I came home from that time away, I found a pool around the corner from my daughter's school, so I'd drop my daughter off and go around the corner for a swim.

I would swim for a bit over half an hour, five days a week – and slowly but surely, my fitness in the pool increased. My eight laps on the first day turned into twenty-eight and then more. My body became a lot stronger. I bought myself gear because I didn't like putting my face in the water, so I had a face mask, snorkel and flippers. It became my quiet time, when I could go into my head and clear my thoughts. Sometimes I would pray, sometimes I found I got clarity about an issue and at other times the ideas came flooding in for what I could do with my Kefi Chicks business.

Find the thing that you love doing. The thing that helps your body move and helps you feel amazing. Many clients tell me that they don't have time to exercise. Basically, that's a goal that's not being set and not being valued, so time is given to some other activity.

What I say to them is, what is the cost to you if you don't exercise? Perhaps getting up a bit earlier each day will help you find a time when you like to exercise. Don't forget it's going to reduce the stress in your life: you'll feel fit, get more stuff done and stop overthinking everything. Before you know it, you're going to be able to find the time to do things.

So many other people tell me that exercising isn't fun and they hate it because they hate sweating. Well, grab a towel and wipe yourself down. Do housework fast, and put the air conditioning on if you need to. These are just excuses and they're keeping you stuck in your story that you can't do this and you can't do that. If you want to be that person and don't make a change, it's not going to be a benefit for you in the long run.

Another thing that people tell me is that when they're exercising it hurts too much, because they get out of breath or their knee/hip/back hurts. Just imagine doing a little bit of exercise every day to build up the capacity in your body. Unless you've got a medical reason not to exercise, everybody should move every day. We already know this.

Small things make a big difference. I remember reading a book about a lady who started walking around her clothesline, walking a bit further every day. Before she knew it, she was walking long distances and her whole body changed. Small steps lead to huge changes.

So often it is our previous experiences, where we think we haven't been successful, that inhibit our actions down the track. We feel like we have failed ourselves, so the negative self-talk becomes louder and louder – we stop doing anything which will lead towards the desired goal. We just give up on ourselves, and we lose our freedom and inspiration – we lose our kefi.

My previous experiences included a serious health scare in 2015 when a routine pap smear turned into something serious. I was told I had abnormal cells, which led to a visit to a specialist where I was told I had stage 1 cancer and needed a full hysterectomy right away. Keep having those regular check-ups!

I took my time with my recuperation and held back from getting into regular exercise. After I got the all clear at my two year check-up, things changed. I trained as a Greek Dance Fitness instructor and I started my daily hour-long walking regime. The pounds of pain started to fall away from my body; I couldn't believe how simple it was.

Stop and review for a moment. What if all of those so-called failures were part of something much larger? They are part of providing you feedback on what works and what does not. I follow the KISS principle of life: 'Keep it simple, sweetie'. Focus on the here and now rather than fast tracking too far into the future. Then just do it! Only do that – nothing else.

Clear your clutter; the clutter in your physical space reflects the clutter of your mind. A clear space will give you the chance to clear your mind and focus on what is important. You are in charge of your mind and your results. You have all the resources that you need in you right now — you are enough and you can succeed. Remember you are doing the best that you can every day with the resources you've got. You are amazing and you can do it.

What is it that you want? Setting some goals is a great place to start to become fitter, stronger and leaner. Quieten your mind and do things that you enjoy; you can easily get it all done when you set your mind to it. Switch on and get it done in the simplest way possible.

Three actions that you can take as a result of reading Kefi Fit:

1) Attend a Greek Dance Fitness class. If you can't do that, put your favourite Greek song on and dance around the lounge room. Nothing like a good Greek song to get your kefi flowing, your hips swaying and your body grooving.

2) Try a new activity that is part of Kefi Fit. Is it walking, swimming, weights, going to fitness classes at a gym, joining a walking club or parkrun group? I find that if I've got music on when I'm going walking, it's much easier to get further along. Start with a simple goal and commitment to change one thing, such as a walk every day. Before you now it you will be feeling better, fitter and stronger.

3) Grab a friend or a family member and explore the possibilities of what you can do together; if you've got a person coming along on the right journey with you, it becomes a commitment and you're more likely to succeed.

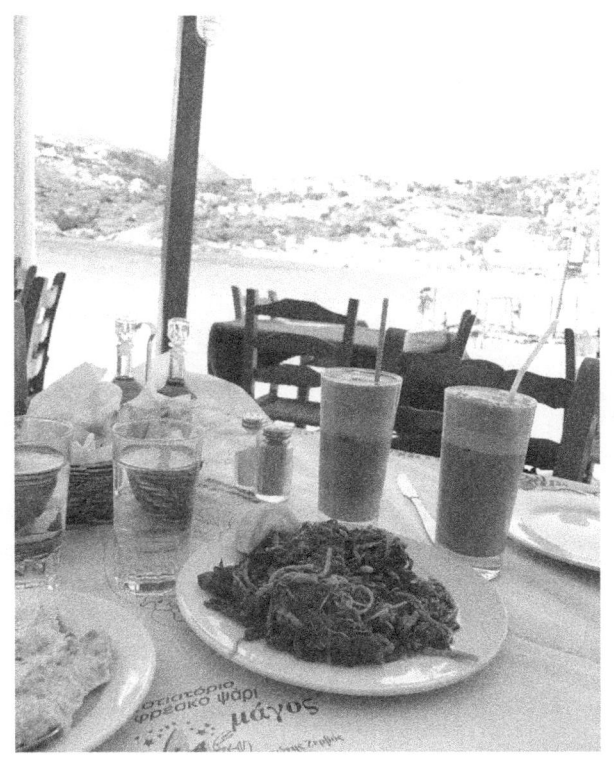

Chapter 10

Kefi Feast

'Seek not good from without, seek it from within.'
— **Epictetus, philosopher**

'Let food be thy medicine and medicine be thy food.'
— **Hippocrates, physician**

Food is central in Greek culture and traditions. Growing up Greek, there's always food around. Food for celebrations, for happy times, for sad times, for when you are hungry and for when you are not. So how do you monitor your eating patterns as a Good Greek Girl?

I can't remember a time when I was growing up when there wasn't food on the table when people were around – family, friends and sometimes even strangers. My mother would tell a story from her childhood, how my grandfather would often come home at night with three or four extra people and the food had already been dished up; the family had to re-plate and share the food for it to go around and to stretch to the guests.

The Greek word *'filoxenia'* means hospitality and generosity of spirit. In ancient Greece this was a high ranking value where great respect was passed on from host to guest. A friend could drop by at any time and be greeted with hospitality, food, drink and a bath. The friend in return responded with courtesy, grace and politeness.

A Kefi Feast is a wonderful thing. A Kefi Feast is where you're offered a range of things, like on a smorgasbord or a banquet, and you get to taste all the flavours. There are many flavours that connect you straight away to Greek culture, traditions and heritage. Straight away I'm sure that you thought of lemon, oregano and mint. Those lemon potatoes that melt in your mouth, which you have with oven-cooked lamb, are bound to evoke a special memory every time. What about the *yemista* (stuffed vegetables) made by your *yiayia* or your mother that has you salivating, or dolmades with a side of Greek yoghurt, and all your other favourite Greek food?

A Kefi Feast is where mothers and grandmothers are at their best. Food and feeding people is an entire experience, from shopping for the freshest ingredients to coming together to make and create the food with a deep love which is part of the flavour. Food made with love is so much more tasty and satisfying.

Eating the food is an event in itself. There's the placement of the guests around the table in just the right spot, then the dramatic arrangement of the platters of food on the table, the savouring of the flavours and the flattery of the cooks. Lastly, there is the ceremonial serving of the dessert. In my family, if it was a birthday cake or something that required serving the job was often given to me. Cutting each piece and being able to serve the cake upright on a plate was a valued skill for us.

As Good Greek Girls, we all know that it's tradition to be able to cook and provide for the family. The kitchen is pivotal to the whole family – this is where the action is, and where the heart and soul of the Greek family comes from.

Nothing is ever done in small measures. Often, I would look at a recipe in a regular recipe book, and make some biscuits where you make twenty-four. Not in my Greek family. It would need to be 224 biscuits before it was even considered remotely enough. Nothing like a *koulouraki* (biscuit) to have next to your coffee as you chat with your mother or your grandmother or any other visitors that came to the home. Large-scale biscuit recipes required several hands to be able to roll out the biscuits, which could take a few hours as you waited for them to cook in the oven.

Food is the connection. Food is good for our soul. It's one of the most obvious connections to our traditions and culture.

Around a Kefi Feast there's also some behaviours that you get to see. There's always enjoyment and laughter — and sometimes there's a few loud voices and a few angry words, as people debate the latest politics. It's where you find out the latest family news, things to celebrate or offer sympathy and understanding towards.

There is no doubt that the Mediterranean diet is indeed exceptionally healthy. There's lots of talk about how it can benefit your health and your waistline. There are always green vegetables such as *vlita* (amaranth greens), spinach and *horta* (boiled greens), with zucchini or green beans as a staple. The bitter greens are served with vinegar or lemon and olive oil. Are you salivating thinking about them? Slow cooking was invented by the Greeks — lamb in the oven done a number of different ways, perhaps in a tomato salsa, served with *avgolemono* (egg and lemon) or marinated with lemon and oregano.

When you are happier, it is easier to be mindful about what you are putting into your mouth. It's easier to decide on the healthier options and limit what goes in your mouth. Not only is the Mediterranean diet a tasty way to eat, drink and live, but it's also a sustainable way to reduce disease-causing inflammation and maintain a healthy weight.

The opposite of all this is that you fear food and you say to yourself, 'Should I be eating this? Oh my gosh, this is just a naughty treat, but I'm going to have it anyway.' There's a real lack of enjoyment around food and a severe lack of connection to your body as you're eating.

When you're self-aware of what you're eating, you'll find things a lot easier. The celebration component that comes with a Kefi Feast is super simple. Adhering to the KISS principle, start by enjoying whatever you are eating. Eat because you are hungry, keep it packed full of flavour and make it with love. Then take the time to sit and enjoy your food. Eat mindfully and with your eyes.

In a Greek household, the kitchen is the hub of the home. One place where kefi is most often observed is around the dinner table, with sometimes large and boisterous family meals. Food is central to Greek family life. There's no doubt about that. Where there is food, there is family. They are interconnected in complex ways.

Looking back over my childhood, my biggest memories involves food. At Christmas, the whole family would get together. My mother was one of six children; they had wives or husbands and everybody had at least three children. My grandmother's sister married my grandfather's brother, so they had four children and they also had husbands and most had children. Then there was my grandmother's brother, who also had children and they'd all come along as well.

All the family was represented, so we're talking forty people minimum. Quite often there would be a number of other family friends who would also be with their partners or their children and a gaggle of grandchildren and so on. It was always loud and fun, with groups of people getting together: cousins aged in the same age bracket, the mothers hanging out together in the kitchen preparing the food and the fathers hanging outside.

Everybody contributed to the amazing array of food because there were too many people for one cook to manage.

Chapter 10 Kefi Feast

Everybody had their speciality. My mother's specialty was to bring the spanakopita (spinach pie). She had it down to a fine art. She had a special way of making her own pastry; the inside of the spanakopita was done in the same way, she used the same spinach, silver beet and cheese, as well as the same hand technique, always made in a round dish and was always cut and served in a certain way.

One year my mother nearly didn't take a spanakopita to a family function and one of my cousins turned around and said to her, 'If you hadn't brought it, it would be like being in a pub with no beer,' which she was particularly chuffed about.

My aunt's speciality was something different and another aunt brought a different thing. There was always at least five different meats: ham, turkey, chicken, pork, lamb, beef, you name it, it was there.

Add a lot of salad and the table would groan under the weight of it all — sometimes it didn't all fit.

And then moving on to dessert, where we also had the same thing going on. Of course there were *kourambiedes* (shortbread covered in icing sugar), *koulouria* (biscuits often with sesame seeds on top) and *melomakarona* (biscuits dipped in honey). All of them were firm family favourites to be had with your tea or coffee, if you could fit it in.

And as the family grew and some of the husbands and wives weren't Greek, the food on the table evolved a little bit as well: we included things like pavlova, cheesecake or trifle into the mix, going together with the *karidopita* (walnut cake) or other things such as the *kourambiedes*, which were always a treat for special occasions such as weddings.

Caring for one's family is a great calling and cooking for others is a ministry. It's a homage to the women in my family who taught us to cook so much. *Paximadia*, *amigdalota*, *tarama*, tzatziki, *yemista*, *soutzoukakia* — you name it, there's a whole range of things that we all love to cook now. They all have a connection to our family kitchen from generations before us; it brings us closer to the traditions, culture and to our heritage.

When I was staying home one year with my then-baby daughter, my mother came up with an idea to create a family cookbook and she was trying to work out how to get it typed up. At that time, she didn't have a computer and was not quite sure how to use one, so I offered to type up the family cookbook of favourite recipes. We started with the recipes from my grandmother and her sister, which were standard in the family, and everybody wanted a copy. We converted them from Greek to English, because not that many in the family were able to read Greek anymore. This cookbook, a homage to my family of favourite recipes, has become a tradition to cook from. It's sought after by friends and many other extended family members.

It is a celebration of our connection. It's a celebration of our culture, traditions and heritage. It's a legacy for future generations, so that they too can cook the recipes and have a connection with the family. The family originated in Greece in the early 1900s. What I learnt from my family is that the connection of food, the connection of a Kefi Feast, is pivotal for a happy life. It brings people together and deepens connection and love.

The flavours of Greece soothe and nurture the soul. All of the recipes are served with flavours and aromas of stories. My *yiayia* and *papou* came to Australia at a time when there weren't so many Greeks, particularly in our small town of Hobart.

Chapter 10   Kefi Feast

My grandmother wasn't a brilliant cook when she arrived in Australia. She was eighteen and often helped with the animals back on her island home, rather than helping her mum in the kitchen. She had a bit of an idea, and certainly didn't go hungry by any stretch of the imagination.

When my grandmother's sister arrived in Australia after marrying my grandfather's brother, that's when the two of them got together and started learning more and more about cooking. There's lots of recipes in the cookbook that are Australian. There's a shortbread given to her by a neighbour, Christmas pudding, fruitcake, minced pies, and other things that are definitely not on the traditional Greek menu. They are, however, firm family favourites together with the other expected treats.

More importantly, they also became part of our family Kefi Feast on a regular basis because of the connection to when they came from Greece, learning new recipes from the ladies they met in Australia. During the war, my grandmother and my aunt would bake *kourambiedes* (Greek shortbread covered in icing sugar) and they had to really beg, borrow and steal all of the icing sugar. They used to sell the *kourambiedes* at the city hall to raise money for the war effort in the early days.

So many people tell me that they get stressed around food when it comes to family. There is confusion over the relationship with food, family and overeating. Reducing the stress around you assists you to make a good decision. Also, so many people have had the experience when food has been pushed on them, even when they are not hungry, and are expected to eat, as it is rude not to.

Often Greek women take care of others before attending to

their own needs. In learning to be the person who looks after themselves first, making a good decision is a key to changing old patterns. So often, people tell me that they go to a relative's place and if there's food put in front of them they eat it, even if they've had dinner and are not hungry.

It's difficult to be rude because when somebody offers you food, it's from a place of *filoxenia* (hospitality), which is a really important concept in the Greek culture. To refuse is impolite.

Other clients have said to me, 'I medicate with food, how can I stop that? I've got this negative relationship with food.' Delving back to when it all started is a great way to explore this habit. Focusing on it too deeply may find you eating more at times; tune into your feelings and let your body show you what it needs.

Perhaps sometimes it's worth connecting with family when there's no meal. Or to really look at what it is that you plan to eat. Take some food with you that you know you can eat. Take a Greek salad and dress it later; control how much dressing and oil is on it. Or go and enjoy the food. Eat without feelings of guilt. Scheduling times with your family to share a meal, to rekindle love and connection or to enhance it, is key.

Kefi Family, that Column of Strength that is pivotal to all relationships around you, is connected to Kefi Feast as well. Eating well, nourishing your body and doing it with kefi, surrounded by people who love and are connected with you, is going to help you have a very good connection with your body. Having a relationship with yourself and knowing what food serves you best is essential.

I know that I have a problem with ice cream. It takes me back to my childhood, when Mum would take us out on a Sunday

Chapter 10 Kefi Feast

afternoon. She would take us to the wharf: we'd walk around and there would be Mr Whippy or the Dairy Queen, my favourite soft serve ice cream. I can still see it now in front of me and taste the creamy, smooth ice cream – it takes me to that happy place. I used to be able to eat a tub of ice cream without too many problems, especially when I was feeling a bit low. I have been known to put the ice cream in the microwave to soften!

When I said to myself I just don't eat ice cream any more, then ice cream was taken out of the zone where I needed to medicate myself. That's why being able to understand how your feelings connect with certain foods can make a huge difference. I now don't even look at ice cream.

Family celebrations and get-togethers are an essential part of life. The word 'control' is often used around food. 'I can't control myself, I can't control what I put in my mouth, I can't control the food that they put in front of me.'

That's basically an excuse. There's no need to be rude, to not eat food, unless you know that you're allergic to it. Perhaps there are ways of being polite and just have a few mouthfuls – acknowledge that you're tasting the food and go from there.

The focus thus far has been on food; there is another way to view the Kefi Feast. Imagine your life is in front of you with a smorgasbord of offerings. There is more peace and happiness in your life. Food is a way to connect more fully to yourself and with others.

A Kefi Feast ensures that you see what life has to offer and you take the opportunity to go for it. Take the chance to make a change by sampling what you wish to try out. If you are content to live a small life with a dampened soul, then you may find that when you reflect over your life you'll have regrets. You are sitting at the banquet of life and you can sample everything before you decide on what you want more of.

Explore the possibilities to live a life filled with kefi. It is in this way that you will find what you are looking for. You can achieve those things that you have always dreamt of; you recognise what it is you truly want and then you give yourself permission to enjoy the fruits of your labour. Life is a feast; you can be on a perpetual diet or you can enjoy every mouthful. You can sample all that life has to offer or you can deny yourself. The choice is yours.

Three actions you can take as a part of reading Kefi Feast:

1) Cook your favourite meal prepared by your mum or *yiayia* and enjoy it. Go through the old recipe books if you have access to them, or google some Greek recipes.

2) Journal what beliefs have you picked up from your family about food, how much you eat and where you share food. What is your Kefi Feast? Do you eat everything on your plate when you are not hungry? Do you feed your emotions or do you feed your body?

3) Treat yourself to a night out with friends or family at a Greek restaurant. Order food that can easily be shared. Dips, *tiropitas*, *yiros* and so on. Go and enjoy your food. *Kali orexi*!

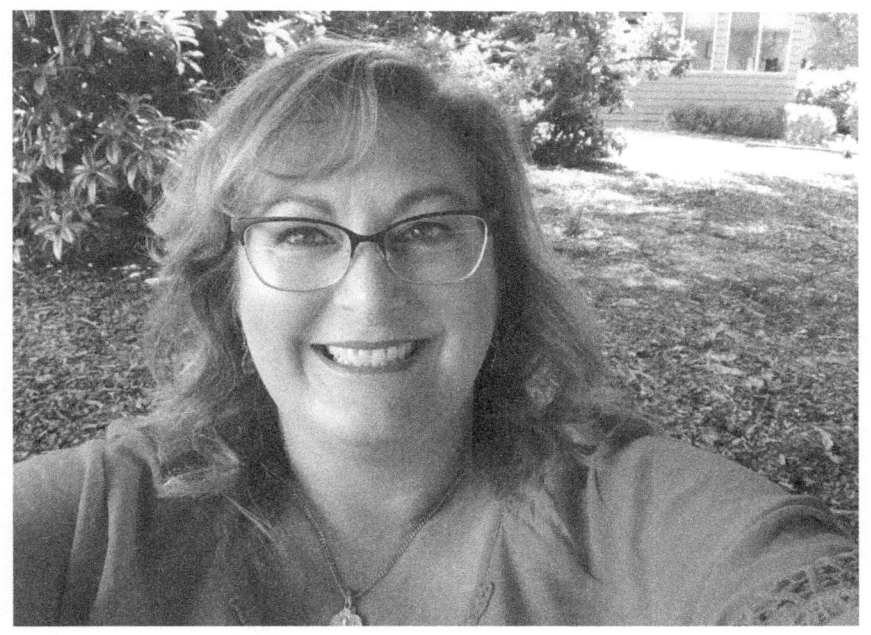

Chapter 11

Kefi Flame

'Love is composed of a single soul
inhabiting two bodies.'
— **Aristotle, philosopher**

'At the touch of love everyone becomes a poet.'
— **Plato. philosopher**

Experiencing a deep, fulfilling, happy relationship with someone can bring such joy. However, if your core needs are not met, it can be harrowing and painful, taking years to get over.

Kefi Flame is all about passion: someone or something that lights you up to be amazing and to reach your full potential. A flame is something that burns bright and illuminates the way. When your Kefi Flame is burning bright you possess an inner glow; there is something about you that others are drawn to. It is all about your inner kefi shining bright for everyone to see. It can be part of a deep fulfilling relationship and it can also represent the inner you that is passionate and purposeful.

This relationship starts with yourself and then moves into other relationships around you. When you are ignited with the joy of life and you pursue a career that you love, it is easy to illuminate your way with your kefi. It all starts with you: what you do and why you do it.

This Column of Strength is about so much more than the obvious. Kefi Flame is about igniting yourself — from that place of illumination, you can see a relationship with a partner or husband that is more than any other relationship you have ever experienced. For some people already in a relationship, it is about experiencing a deeper and more passionate connection. Understanding your personal relationships with your loved one, — your other half, your soulmate, your twin flame, whatever you want to call them — can validate you in a way like no other relationship. Becoming aware of who you are, connecting with your culture, heritage and traditions add to that.

As you explore your Columns of Strength you can comprehend who you are and what you believe to be true for you – so your true self can emerge from the shadows. As a Good Greek Girl it is so easy to hide your true self and forget who you really are, becoming immersed in people pleasing, not dealing fully with your emotions, eating when you are not hungry, putting yourself last, and only doing something if you can do it perfectly.

When young people get into relationships, it is possible to observe the types of relationships they've grown up around. If all they have seen are relationships that are controlling or abusive (verbally, physically or both), this can impact on how they behave around their loved ones. If they see things that are dysfunctional, the tendency is to see this as the norm – it becomes the marker for what their relationship should be. They do not possess the skills and resources they need.

Having a Kefi Flame relationship is like no other. Imagine how you feel in this relationship, the one that starts with you and then encompasses your partner. Communication happens on a deeper level, as you can talk about anything and everything. You are connected on a spiritual level through your Kefi Faith. You have shared values and beliefs when it comes to Kefi Family, Kefi Friends, Kefi Future and Kefi Fortune. You enhance each other and complement each other at the same time.

Know that you are all-important. When you are having a love affair, so to speak, with yourself, that is when you do things that other people would conceive to be selfish – such as taking time out for yourself, doing what you want to do without others, taking yourself out for a delicious meal, going to bed early and nourishing your body in ways that are going to keep you fit, strong and healthy — and keep your kefi alive. It is so much more than the basic everyday things that you do.

When you have a full-on Kefi Flame relationship with yourself, it means that you attract what you give out. It means that the people around you mirror you and are like you. That person who's attracted to you is going to be amazing if they haven't come into your life as yet. On the flip side, if you already have a partner or husband, imagine the deeper level of love that you can develop because of your greater understanding of who you are and what you stand for. By becoming the best version of yourself, you will bring out the best in others.

However, I offer a warning at this point. When you shake your tree, you also shake the tree of the people already in your life; you may find that you are in for a bumpy ride for a bit while everything assimilates and integrates. The 'C' word — Change — can be pretty confronting for some people, so they are challenged and can rock the boat. If this happens to you, know that you are on the right track. You are bringing a new energy into your relationship, even though it may not be embraced by others the way that you are embracing it.

The 'journey to love', as my friend calls it, can be very empowering. Many Kefi Chicks that I speak to are coming out of unsatisfying relationships with a husband or a partner. Some make the mistake of going straight into another relationship without doing any personal development or reflection. They find they are back where they started, with the same sort of unsatisfying experience.

Taking the time to complete the full healing process, to let go of what happened in the past relationship, will empower you so much. When you do that, you will attract someone amazing and have a very new, exciting Kefi Flame relationship — if that is what you want for yourself.

The opposite of this is that you can end up alone and disconnected from yourself, feeling bitter about men and how things work. Your Kefi Flame is almost out and this requires you to pay some attention to what lights you up. Is your job an unfulfilling experience and you struggle to get out of bed in the morning? Do you get along with your colleagues? Do you have a demanding, unappreciative boss? What isn't working for you in your life?

Now is the time to take action. What have you got to lose if you do?

What I know for sure is that when you've done the healing — when you've cleared the past and love yourself in a way that is full and connected — you'll attract that big love into your life. You will find that person who you'll perhaps spend the rest of your life (or at least some quality time) with. It may start with flirtation, getting to know them on a deeper friendship level first. It may come out of the blue and creep up on you.

That doesn't mean that there won't ever be any issues. It doesn't mean that life will be like living in a castle with a king and you're the queen. That's not how it works.

In a Kefi Flame relationship, your core needs are met. It means that you're certain about the other person in the relationship, because there's excellent communication and there's no doubt, fear and control. You know that you are loved, because you're communicating that and you're speaking the love language of your partner. They just get you and you get them.

You grow together; you bring out the potential in each other, always boosting each other up rather than tearing each other down. It's not a competition and it allows you to keep your own personality and independence, but you come together as one at times.

There is no doubt everyone needs to know they are loved. Everyone needs love in their life in some way, shape or form. Self-love is where it starts, where you are kind to yourself and gentle with your self-talk. You are empowered to be whole and free, which leads to an inspired life.

The romantic idea of love can cause issues, because if you think of the prince and princess riding off into the sunset, living happily ever after without doing any work, communicating or making allowances for each other, that's where things come undone.

Whether you're trying to understand your relationship with another person or you're trying to understand the tension in a relationship, you need to understand what you mean when you say the word 'love'. Understanding your values and your belief system around love will set you up for the future.

One of the things which has most helped me understand what I mean about love, and how to evaluate how I'm doing loving myself and any potential partner in my future, is looking at the various words for love in Greek. We have the word '*agape*', which is the one that is the most common, is love that you open up to. We have the word '*eros*' which means sexual passion, '*erotas*' which means intimate love, and '*filia*' which is love of a friend.

Having a deep relationship either with yourself or another person is indeed one of the most amazing things in your life. So many people settle in an attempt to control the other person in their romantic relationship. Imagine how it could be if you loved unconditionally, without judgement, criticism, fear or a sense of lack? Imagine how it would feel having a relationship where there is acceptance, honour and respect. Just take the time to reflect.

In my past relationships, I settled in so many ways. I attracted people who couldn't connect with me in the way that I wanted, because I was trying to control things all the time.

There were times when I've had partners say that I was behaving like their mother, that I was trying to control every word and every need. That was certainly not my intention; I just wanted things to be better, I wanted things to be *more*.

My first boyfriend was Greek and I thought that we were going to get married one day. I was seventeen and he was eighteen. Even to this day people still tell me that they had expected us to get married back then. In so many ways I played the victim in that relationship, because I was always in tears – I always felt lost and fearful that we would break up.

I found that I was not quite sure how I should behave, because Good Greek Girls didn't do certain things and it was always a challenge to behave the way I wanted. I had no idea about relationships and how I should behave – it was all a learning curve and in a lot of ways, that part of that relationship was not so great. I can remember my sister and friends saying, 'What do you put up with it for?'

Fast forward into the future to when I got married: not long into my marriage I saw that I had married a similar person to my first boyfriend. Also, the behaviours that I exhibited were very

Chapter 11   Kefi Flame

similar. There were always tears and I always blamed myself with what had gone wrong and what was going on around me. I beat myself up so often about the way I looked and I spent time in the pantry, eating everything even when I wasn't hungry.

I was the one who needed to change — to stop being the Good Greek Girl who didn't get her needs met and was very confused and fearful.

Learning to love myself unconditionally — which means finding happiness in a relationship based on friendship and individual freedom without restriction — was an empowering moment for me. Having understanding and forgiveness, and the joy of being happy on my own, has really given me the power to do more than I ever imagined. Becoming a Kefi Chick and being the flame I want in my own life is pure gold. I do what is best for me, so that I can be more. I live my life with my children and give to them unconditionally. And the relationship I've always dreamed of with someone someday (and the signs are there that something is developing) has been the icing on the cake.

It didn't happen overnight, but it did happen. I unpacked what lights me up, I immersed myself in passion projects and I inspired both myself and others.

Once I took the step to free myself from my marriage and look hard at myself, to be honest about what was going on, that's when change happened. It's when the kefi happened. Bit by bit, I was hardly aware of what was going on until one day I stopped to reflect. That's when I noticed what had changed; the small things all added up to a massive change in how I lived my life.

I found that when I looked into all of my Columns of Strength

– knowing what makes me happy, what is fulfilling and what is powerful for me – that's when things took off and I achieved so much more than I ever envisaged. I viewed each Column of Strength and I reviewed my goals and dreams. I looked at how I wanted my home to be, how I wanted to be as a person. I looked at how I could be that person I always aspired to be, so I could inspire others.

The size of my Kefi Flame grows every day. It also illuminates the way for others.

I want no Kefi Chicks left behind. I'm taking you all with me so that you too can have a better life and have that relationship with yourself first and foremost – and then with another person. The person that may become your husband – maybe he is your husband already. You can enhance the relationships that you have right now; you can be more than what you have had in the past. It is a wonderful thing.

One book that really helped me understand the breakdown of my marriage was *The Five Love Languages* by Gary Chapman. I understood what my love languages were and I looked at what my ex-husband's were – and I had an epiphany. This was why we had difficulty communicating. Communication is key in every relationship. So is knowing what you believe in and what you prefer. Consider how you can make it better for the other person, by speaking to them in a way that they understand.

On top of the five love languages, there's also learning styles. Know if your partner is a visual learner, an auditory learner (learn by listening), a kinaesthetic learner (learn by doing) and or an auditory digital person where they do a lot of headspace thinking. It is a communication game-changer!

Chapter 11 Kefi Flame

Knowing how to speak to them in the language that works for them is really powerful. You can communicate in a way that shows that you get them, so understanding this is going to be amazing. Communication is key. When you speak your mind in a respectful manner without causing pain and heartache, this is where you empower yourself and your partner — and the only result possible is that you have a Kefi Flame relationship that is outstanding.

So many people tell me that they don't think they're loveable. The way forward in this is personal development. You can either do it by yourself — online, you can find all the things that you need — or you can get yourself a coach, a counsellor or some professional person to assist you to go deeper. In either case, you review your values and your belief system and all those defining moments that have caused you to think the way that you do.

Let's bust those myths. Good Greek Girls can and should be more; they have a right to be more. Often people say to me, 'No one would be interested in someone my size.' Let me tell you, I can remember saying those same things.

One day a few years ago, I said, 'I reckon that I can attract someone who isn't interested in size, who'll be able to see me for who I am.' That very night, I met somebody. Which is another story for another day. I was amazed that it was possible at the time.

It is possible for you to attract people who are not interested in body size or shape. They're interested in the person and the connection, so if you look around, you'll find that lots of people have these sorts of relationships.

The other one that I love so much is, 'There are no good men out there.' I would ask, 'Where are you looking?' I'm actually not a fan of online dating, because I don't believe that it gives you the opportunity to connect with people and to get an impression. Many people have said to me that they wish that they could do a *proxenio* (marriage introduction/setup) and have the opportunity to meet somebody that way.

Three actions you can take as a part of reading Kefi Flame:

1) Journal what love is to you. Look at what you can do to bring more love into your relationship. Quite often we have rules about what love is, what it looks like and what the other person has to do to show they love you. What five things do you need to feel loved?

2) Stop waiting for the knight in shining armour. Buy yourself those red roses. Romance yourself, light candles, watch a romantic movie – you get the idea.

3) Get out there; nothing is going to happen if you sit at home alone. Join a club, go to a dance, walk a dog on the beach. You never know who you're going to meet and where you are going to meet them. Watch out for the signs. I know people who have met at church, at a dance, at a gym, walking, through other people. Be open to the opportunities.

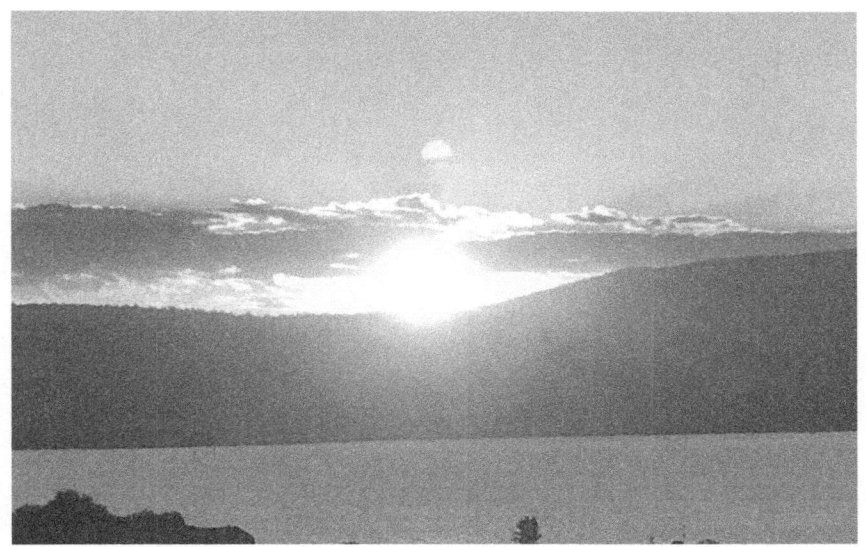

Chapter 12

Kefi Life

'The aim of the wise is not to secure pleasure
but to avoid pain.'
— **Aristotle, philosopher**

'Beware of the barrenness of a busy life.'
— **Socrates, philosopher**

After getting this far, you've worked out what you need for a kefi life. Sometimes you have to go a bit further than you ever expected to get the results that you're looking for. Each and every one of the eight Columns of Strength will give you the power and the courage to make the change that you need to.

Are these the only eight columns? Absolutely not. There are other columns in the Parthenon to keep the whole building standing. But the very front columns, the ones you see in those famous pictures, are the ones that are going to hold you up and keep you going in ways that you never thought possible.

When you live a kefi-filled life, you feel happy and fulfilled. You see the smiling faces of the people in your family, your home and all around you. You hear loving words of kindness and you can feel appreciated and fulfilled – and you just have the inner knowledge that you're doing the right thing.

With a kefi life, everything is easy and wonderful. That's not to say that there will never be times when there are challenges and or things you need to work on. That's part of life.

Sometimes things may seem boring, so things get shaken a little bit. The most amazing thing about a kefi life is that you'll get stuff done. You'll create the space to have a great relationship, enjoy your home, go on holidays, get fitter and healthier, lose that weight, get that job, start the business. You are lit from within and you know intrinsically that you can get stuff done and make it happen for you.

You're going to feel successful and wealthy, inside and out.

When your inner body matches your outer body and the experiences around you, you're in a state of harmony – and that's the aim of the game.

Good Greek Girls know that they need to show appreciation and gratitude. Some of the myths of being a Good Greek Girl can be very challenging and seem to focus on the negative. In actual fact, it is the opposite when a Good Greek Girl knows her life is good. She knows when to be appreciative and when to see the good everywhere.

Life without kefi is like food without flavour. We are not meant to live a bland life. I had a grade 4 student once who told me about how people are colours. I turned and said to him, 'Oh, so what colour am I?' He said (and I was called Mrs M at the time), 'Well, you know how there are beige people? Mrs M, you are not beige. You definitely are not beige.'

I know some colourless people who are living without kefi and it shows.

With the kefi in your life, there's no way that you can be a beige person. Or like in *My Big Fat Greek Wedding*, when the father of Nia Vardalos' character turns and says that the in-laws are like dry toast.

In actual fact, when you don't know how to have a kefi-filled life, perhaps your life is a bit like dried toast. Isn't it going to be great when you move on and change it? Because living as a negative Nancy or a sad sack Sally is not on. We are not going to live our life in fear of not being good enough. Let's embrace our kefi and live a colourful life with no regrets.

When asking Greek speakers what kefi means, they say that it means you're joyful, spirited, passionate and happy in general. That you love life. This is more descriptive than what the definition of kefi is according to the language translator. But it still doesn't tell you the whole story.

Kefi is a way of life. In general, kefi is the way Greeks express their positive emotions. It is the art of being in a happy mood and letting that shape your experiences. It's possible to be in a good mood even if times are tough. In fact, this offers a healthy and balanced approach to living life. We have the glass half-empty people and the glass half-full people, and then we have the people where it doesn't really matter if it's half-full or half-empty because it's just life.

What we want to do is be able to embrace all of life and see both sides. We want to live a balanced and peaceful life, because that's what it's all about.

The true feeling of kefi is tested even when times are tough. With it you can come out the other side. You know that this too shall pass, just like you know that the sun will rise in the morning.

Every time I know that I'm about to make something happen or make a big change, I know I'm being tested. Expect to feel the tests and to experience this. It could be people, or a circumstance, or wanting to start a business. Or you change your workspace and suddenly all your technology doesn't work.

When you know and understand that things get challenged, it can make a difference. Just see them for what they are; don't obsess over them and overthink them. Just let it go.

There are different ways that Greeks express kefi. There are actual tangible moments that we all witness and experience ourselves. It's the simplicity and joy of sharing a meal with loved ones and eating delicious food. We can find our kefi when dancing and creating music. Mostly, people who have truly found their kefi are able to relax and enjoy the good moments of life no matter what.

Sitting down and reflecting how far I'd come on my own personal journey this year was exceptionally empowering. I was able to see that through thick and thin I've been able to stick to my guns while exploring the world of kefi: the world where I live and how I found my joy and inner peace. People tell me that I now glow – it's easy to see that the experiences are past and no longer evident by just looking at my face.

The journey of self-discovery has been empowering and enlightening. This didn't happen on my own and I've had a series of mentors and coaches who have helped me along the way. For a while I tried to do it on my own, and there were times when I was over-giving to everybody else, being over-responsible and giving to everybody but myself.

And it wasn't until I started investing in myself fully by starting to attend courses that things changed. There are many online and physical courses that you can do. There are books you can read to motivate you to change your behaviour.

It's time to sit down and reflect what it is you truly want for yourself.

The spirit of kefi is something that anyone can have. The immigrants from Greece who travelled to other places such as Australia, the United Kingdom, Canada and the United States have kept this feeling alive. In fact, everyone who has ever visited Greece is surely impacted by the effect kefi had on them while in Greece.

You can step into a Greek restaurant in any part of the world and you know what's on the menu. You know there will be Greek music in the background, there will be a twinkle in the eye of the waiter and if the music is just right and the kefi is there, there will be dancing.

Dancing is where it's at. Dancing the dance of life, dancing the Zorba or the Kalamatiano or any of those other dances, is how we traverse life. We dance in circles when we dance in Greek dances and the circle of life goes around and around. There is no need for a partner and everyone gets to join in.

It's how it's supposed to be and how it will always be.

Often people say to me, 'This can't happen for me, I can't live a kefi life. Nothing is going to change, I'm not good enough.' All that negative Nancy talk.

You can be the person who says that they aren't good enough or you can take a chance on life and make it happen. Get some coaching. Re-read *The Kefi Effect* and scribble all over it – follow the steps, take the recommended actions and trust the process.

'This is all too hard,' is something I hear way too often. 'It's so hard to lose weight, it's so hard to change, it's so hard to make friends, to find a husband, blah blah blah.'

If you look back on your life, what are you going to be grateful for? What are you grateful for right now? What are you focusing on that is good? Because as we know, where attention goes is where the energy flows.

If you keep focusing on the negative Nancy stuff, nothing is going to change. Nancy only sees the negative; she has a negative attitude and expects that things will not work out for her, as she considers herself unworthy or not good enough. If you look at all the other things happening in your life, you're going to find that you attract the people in your life who need to help you grow stronger. You attract what you put out. When you raise your awareness to this, you can begin to change your story and be more.

What's on your bucket list that you really want to achieve? The biggest question of all that people ask me is, 'How do I find my kefi?' Take small steps every day, review your Column of Strength and take the chance. Apply for that promotion; join a club, go to where you'll find your tribe; go to church, renew your spirit and faith. Choose to be more; take on everything that you possibly can. Take the step forward, life is waiting for you. What are you waiting for?

Raise your awareness; catch yourself during a moment of kefi and anchor it. If you know that going to a Greek Dance Fitness class is going to raise your kefi and help you shift all of that negative stuff in your body, then go do that.

Have you reviewed your Columns of Strength and looked at what it is that you can do to improve right now? Have you committed to changing things and followed through with the suggestions at the end of each chapter?

What can you do to help yourself? What things do you want to change or build on right now? Build that strength — know

Chapter 12   Kefi Life

that you have the courage and capacity right now to do all the things. You can leave victimhood and blame behind and take a step in the other direction. Are you ready? Because you can do it right now.

Have faith that you can change, believe in yourself and achieve. I'm here to help you. Most importantly, what are you going to do to celebrate? Celebrate your wins along the way. You can come and party with me any time you like. Stop and immerse yourself in the process to know who you are and renew your identity – to celebrate your culture, traditions and heritage. Go to that local Greek festival down the road that you keep saying you're going to attend. Have a souvlaki, have a gyro, have some *loukoumades*. Enjoy them – know that this is part of who you always were and always will be. You will only succeed.

What are you waiting for?

Go out and have that kefi life.

Life starts with you.

Afterword

Thank you for spending the time delving into the world of kefi. As a Good Greek Girl, life can prove to be confusing and filled with trials and tribulations. I trust you have picked up a few tricks, tips and strategies along the way to build your capacity as a Kefi Chick. Living a life filled with kefi can play such a huge role in how you live your life and how you embrace the opportunities which come your way.

Life immersed in the tradition, heritage and culture of a Greek life can be enriching and wonderful when you're in the right mindset and headspace. It is possible to turn things around – follow the process and do the things that you know will make a difference. Take the time to enjoy your exploration and connection to your Columns of Strength, as they are the keys to living a full and happy life.

Know for sure that you want your children, nieces and girls around you to be clear of the impact of being a Good Greek Girl, living life in a way that is no longer right for young women today.

Create a kefi-filled life full of kindness, empowerment, freedom and inspiration – these are the underlying pillars, the foundations of your Columns of Strength. Small simple steps will bring great change. Take the step.

Glossary

Brain dump	A technique to clear your over-active mind. Write down everything that you're thinking about, all the thoughts that keep popping up, and the conversations you wish you had (or actually had in real life). You are dumping your excess onto paper.
Journal	Journals are written for different purposes. It is a reflective technique which helps us see different points of view, to unpack beliefs and values and see a bigger picture. It can be the stimulus to re-frame your perspective, see things from a different point of view and can help clarify what you really want.
Mind Map	A planning and organisation tool which is excellent for visual people. A central idea is placed in the middle and associated ideas are placed around the page. Images, drawings or words may be placed around the central idea to expand it more fully.
SMART	A goal setting technique which focuses on the specific steps involved in attaining the goal. The acronym stands for Specific, Measurable, Attainable, Realistic and Timed. This technique is often observed as a one page template where the details are recorded and observed.

Vision board   A tool used to help clarify, concentrate and maintain focus on a specific life goal. It is any sort of board or large poster on which you display images that represent whatever you want to be, do or have in your life. Focusing on how you feel when you look at the images provides you with clarity to assist you achieve your goals.

Appendix 1 – Budget Template

	Weekly or fortnightly	Monthly	Yearly
Home expenses			
Phone/internet			
Electricity			
Water			
Mortgage/rent			
Insurance			
Media (e.g. Netflix, Stan, Foxtel)			
Groceries (including alcohol and takeaway)			
Car expenses			
Petrol			
Maintenance			
Insurance			
Repayments			

	Weekly or fortnightly	Monthly	Yearly
School fees/childcare			
Personal expenses			
Toiletries			
Hair			
Clothing			
Gym membership			
Health (doctor, dentist, health insurance, medication, etc.)			
Holidays and travel			
Entertainment			
Gifts			
TOTAL			

Appendix 2 – SMART Goals Template

S	Specific • Keep goals simple • Be clear and detailed	
M	Measurable • Criteria for achieving goal • Easily tracked achievements	
A	Attainable • Keep it appealing • State as if you have already accomplished your goals	
R	Realistic • Keep attainable goals • Believe it can happen	
T	Timely • Reasonable time frame • Feel and sense when it's achieved	

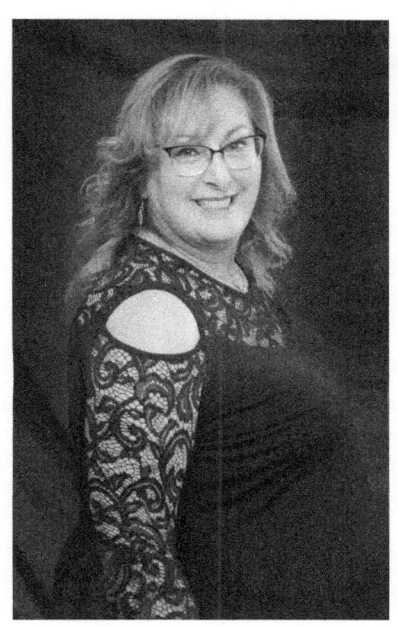

About the Author

Irini has always held a deep love for her Greek background, instilled in her by her parents and grandparents. She loves to travel to Greece and spent time assisting her local Greek community and the Executive Greek Community Committee – and, until 2017, the Estia Festival Committee (Chair in 2016). She also volunteers at St George's Greek Orthodox Church. She loves to dance and has started up Greek Dance Fitness classes for women in her local Greek community.

Irini knows what it is like to live life as a Good Greek Girl – the good and the bad experiences as a result led her to create Kefi Chicks. She experienced divorce, grief and feelings of powerlessness. She had no kefi, no dreams and no hope. She stepped up, took a chance and made a choice to change!

Then she had some life coaching and learnt a lot about herself, her fears and her overwhelm. She finally understood that she was not invisible and certainly mattered. She got her kefi back with her Greek heritage, her community and her faith.

Irini has a background in teaching for over thirty years, is a trained life coach, an NLP practitioner and an experienced party plan consultant. She mentors women around the world to get what they want, build their confidence and get results, to find their kefi again.

Her mission is to support and mentor women to build their kefi, to be a true reflection of who they are! She loves assisting women to create businesses and laying out the simple steps to get it all going.

Now she coaches and mentors women just like you to get it together post-divorce or relationship breakdown, to be proud and empowered rather than losing your identity in who you think you should be passed on from previous generations.

Now she also plans awesome fun-filled adventures for herself, her kids and her Kefi Chick community. Retreat to Greece, did you say?

Email: **irini@kefichicks.com**

Website: **www.kefichicks.com**

www.thekefieffect.com

Free Kefi Bonus

Thank you for reading *The Kefi Effect*! If you loved what you have read, you might like some additional hot tips to find more balance, focus and success in your life. Irini has compiled this FREE Bonus download to assist you with more valuable strategies so you can move forward right now! So many of her clients talk about how difficult it is to find the family, life and work balance and how to focus on the things that matter and are important.

It is ready and available for you to download FREE at:

http://kefichicks.com/bonus/

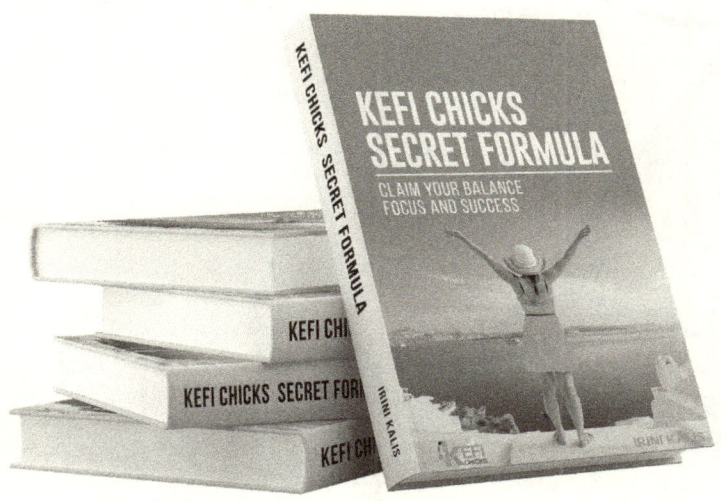

Engage Irini to Speak at Your Next Event!

Irini Kalis is The Kefi Effect Author. A highly sought after speaker, Irini is the creator of the Kefi Chicks movement. She knows what it is like to live life as a Good Greek Girl – the contradiction of this led her to create Kefi Chicks. She implements her 8 Columns of Strength System with clients online and in person at workshops and retreats.

Her mission is to support and mentor women to build their kefi, to be a true reflection of who they are and to be the best woman they can be to positively impact their daughters, nieces, and granddaughters!

Her mission is to support and mentor women to build their kefi, to be a true reflection of who they are and to be the best woman they can be to positively impact their daughters, nieces, and grand daughters!

Irini shares the answers to all of this and more, sharing her wisdom in a variety of media outlets and platforms spreading the Kefi message around the world, assisting Greek women live an empowered life both personally and in their business or career.

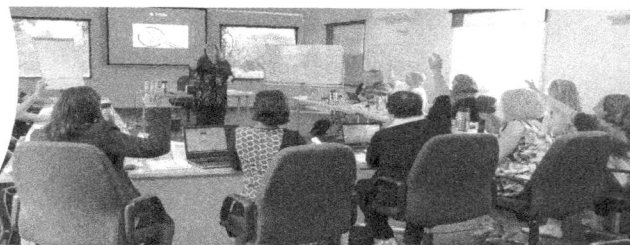

The Kefi Effect
- Flip your life with a touch of kefi
- Bust that Good Greek Girl Myth
- Create your Kefi Reality Quick Shots

Kefi Chick Wisdom
- Create your Acropolis with the 8 Columns of Strength - Kefi Family, Kefi Friends, Kefi Future, Kefi Fortune, Kefi Faith, Kefi Fit, Kefi Feast, Kefi Flame
- Four Pillars for Success
- Where did my Kefi go and how do I find it?

Kefi Chicks Secret Formula
- Create a Kefi filled business Fast Track System
- Technology Tips and Tricks
- Mindset and Communication Mastery in Minutes

Phone: +61 408624129
Email: irini@kefichicks.com
Website: www.kefichicks.com
www.thekefieffect.com